D0255319

THE UNITED STATES UNIFORMED SERVICES OATH OF OFFICE:

"I, Reagan B. Anderson, do solemnly swear (or affirm) that I will support and defend the Constitution of the United States against all enemies, foreign and domestic; that I will bear true faith and allegiance to the same; that I take this obligation freely, without any mental reservation or purpose of evasion; and that I will well and faithfully discharge the duties of the office on which I am about to enter. So help me God."

THE OSTEOPATHIC OATH:

"I do hereby affirm my loyalty to the profession I am about to enter. I will be mindful always of my great responsibility to preserve the health and the life of my patients, to retain their confidence and respect both as a physician and a friend who will guard their secrets with scrupulous honor and fidelity, to perform faithfully my professional duties, to employ only those recognized methods of treatment consistent with good judgment and with my skill and ability, keeping in mind always nature's laws and the body's inherent capacity for recovery.

I will be ever vigilant in aiding in the general welfare of the community, sustaining its laws and institutions, not engaging in those practices which will in any way bring shame or discredit upon myself or my profession. ..."

UNIVERSAL DEATH CARE

A SOLUTION FOR HEALTHCARE IN THE AGE OF ENTITLEMENT

Dr. Reagan B. Anderson

USMC First Reconnaissance Battalion Surgeon (former)

Copyright © 2020 by Dr. Reagan B. Anderson.

All rights reserved. No part of this book may be reproduced in any written, electronic, recording, or photocopying without written permission of the publisher or author. The exception would be in the case of brief quotations embodied in articles or reviews and pages where permission is specifically granted by the publisher or author.

Dr. Reagan B. Anderson/Universal Death Care
Printed in the United States of America

For more information visit www.reaganbanderson.com

Although every precaution has been taken to verify the accuracy of the information contained herein, the author and publisher assume no responsibility for any errors or omissions. No liability is assumed for damages that may result from the use of information contained within.

Universal Death Care/ Dr. Reagan B. Anderson -- 1st ed.

LCCN: 2020902859

ISBN 978-1-7346483-1-7 PAPERBACK EDITION
ISBN 978-1-7346483-0-0 HARDCOVER EDITION
ISBN 978-1-7346483-2-4 EBOOK EDITION

Contents

This book is dedicated to a world filled with healthy, thriving people maximizing their potential.

INTRODUCTION

"If you do not see yourself as part of the problem, you will never see yourself as part of the solution."
- Unknown Author

I WOKE UP WITH 10-out-of-10 pain. I awakened my wife and she drove me to the closest ER, but I felt every bump in the road, every turn, every slight acceleration. The pain soared. When we got to the hospital, I staggered in because my stubborn pride refused anyone's assistance.

I told the nurse, "I am Dr. Anderson and have a surgical abdomen (meaning, 'I need emergent abdominal surgery'). I probably have one or two minutes before I pass out."

They took me back right away, poked and prodded my abdomen, ordered labs for the blood draw, plus a CT scan, with and without contrast. The pain was so bad that I could not open my left eye and my entire face felt like I'd been pricked by thousands of needles—my appendix had ruptured the day before. My belly was full of pus. Into the operating room, out to post-op, then up to the surgical recovery floor. It all happened so quickly. In the middle of the first night, I got out of bed and went for a slow walk down the hallway, trying to keep the circulation flowing so that I wouldn't get a blood clot as well. Then it hit me.

What if I didn't have good insurance? What if I were like countless Americans who have a $5,000-10,000 deductible? What if I was scraping by? If that were the case, then I would not only have to worry about my health, I'd have an added hurdle: how to pay the bills and still have money to put food on the table. Our health care system must adapt to our needs—to worry about money while also fighting back to health is asking too much.

I'm a former Special Forces combat doctor with an impeccable record after two combat deployments to Fallujah, Iraq, and I was reduced to a man who spent the Fourth of July in America curled up in a closet, begging for the fireworks to stop. I spent years as a hypervigilant insomniac, pushing everyone away from my problems. It took me over a decade to rebuild and now I am stronger, wiser, and purpose-driven to change this world for the better. Being a cog in the wheel of the war machine, and a cog in the wheel of a broken medical system in the US, I feel compelled to use all of my experiences to make this world a better place, to strengthen our great country, and to help you understand a little more about war, health care, and our great democracy that is under attack. I took an oath to defend this country against enemies foreign and domestic; this book is an avenue to keep that promise to God and country.

Our world is one that balances health between ideals and realities. Ideally, when someone is in need, the community gives freely and abundantly because we all assume personal accountability. We can take care of ourselves, and when called, we care for each other. We don't ask for receipts. We don't ask for more

"Of the people, by the people, for the people" - Abraham Lincoln

than we need. In reality, that's NOT how it works. It's selfish, even acceptable, to place the onus on others (as it relates to individual health or the collective). To realize these ideals, however, we cannot selfishly consume other people's resources. Luckily, there is a third side to our equation: the issues that bridge into both practice and principle. In the future, will we learn from our mistakes, and finally create a just society filled with individuals who contribute more than they take? We can only live in an abundant world if everyone agrees to take responsibility and chooses to be the change they wish to see in the world.

I am currently a civilian dermatologist practicing in Colorado. Beforehand, I was the doctor to a battalion that was considered to be the Special Forces component of the United States Marine Corps (USMC), First Reconnaissance Battalion (Recon BN). I did two combat deployments to Fallujah, Iraq with Recon BN and then separated from the military. I have a Master of Public Health degree as well as a Master of Christian Studies degree.

My experiences as a combat doctor in Iraq grant me the perspective needed to see the flaws in the medical and military systems. But in doing so, I must acknowledge my heartaches and vulnerabilities. Names and inconsequential details have been changed to protect others' privacy. This is only one side of the story, and we all know that stories have at least three sides: my side, the other side, and the actual "truth."

The truth, like the past, is layered. Please understand that trauma has torn holes in my memory, and I have patched it back together after two deployments to Fallujah. Iraq altered everything about me: what I believed, who I am. Because the memories

"Of the people, by the people, for the people" - Abraham Lincoln

have been overlaid, filed one on top of another, there's no way they're completely accurate. Nothing, including an intact and reliable representation of time, survived the carnage of being a Special Forces combat doctor in war. I think some of my memories are more tangled—a mess of multiple events that my mind has re-recorded as a solitary image, like a double exposure. I would not be surprised if my recollection is factually off base, but I do believe that I have captured the moments, emotions, and ramifications of these events in an honest manner, where the moral of the story is the point, but the facts are off. In other words, I will relay imperfect, true stories, and hopefully, they will illuminate the issues of war and health care with new light.

Also, I would like to first apologize for my language. In an attempt to be as honest as possible I have used the language which supports my mindset and who I was in the moment. I am so sorry if my thought processes are unsettling or vulgar. I need to bring you into that world for a little while, which may be uncomfortable to read because the experiences were painful and inappropriate to live through. Still, war is not pain-free or appropriate—neither is our current health care system.

What does the war in Iraq have to do with the overall discussion of health care in the US? That is a question I have asked myself quite a few times during this process. We all know that the truths of storytelling are universal, and that is why fairy tales are told, why Jesus spoke in parables, and why I am using them here—their applicability is not limited to specific circumstances. My experiences as a combat doc, a civilian doc, and a clinic owner have given me more exposure than most people or doctors have,

"Of the people, by the people, for the people" - Abraham Lincoln

giving me insight into how medicine really works; it is through these lenses that I write and humbly ask you to read it critically, think about it honestly, and then deliberate on finding healthful solutions for our great country.

Yet, perhaps, the hardest truth is this one: after I volunteered to serve in the military, then volunteered to go to war, I had little to no control over my decisions; nevertheless, I am complicit as a small cog in a very big war machine. Similarly, I am a part of American health care delivery and consumption. And, again, while I have little control over anything that transpires within such a system, I choose to participate in it. War and health care are massive beasts that destroy everyone in their path. I feel empowered to change them both.

I hope that my experiences may offer a different perspective than you had before. Maybe, if I am allowed to believe in miracles, this book will inspire you to have a dialogue with someone who has a different viewpoint, someone who will challenge your side—your thoughts, beliefs, and fears on the topics of public health and war. Only when we understand both sides of an issue can we come together to solve it, realizing that we are more alike than different. We are simply human. We want the same things: security, health, and happiness.

Thank you. I am grateful for you all.

Dr. Reagan B. Anderson, First Reconnaissance Battalion
Surgeon (former)

"Of the people, by the people, for the people" - Abraham Lincoln

THE ROADMAP

Chapter 1 – Light Discipline
My introduction to Iraq and your introduction to the necessity for practical, proactive health care. One day, we will all be in need of it.

Chapter 2 – From Left to Right
The concept of universal health care is not a liberal or conservative construct. Arguably, it is the most fiscally conservative and socially responsible way to deliver care—when it is done properly.

Chapter 3 – What Starves a Man Into the Fear of Love and Success?
How do we combat the fear we face in making changes to something as vital as our health care?

Chapter 4 – Coping with the Enemy
Here we discuss how trauma and hurtful experiences have taken Americans down the path to self-sabotaging our health, as well as any chance for universal health care. We need change.

Chapter 5 – Make a Hole!
You and I must approach health care from informed standpoints instead of convenient ignorance. From an open-minded perspective, we can see what works and what doesn't for individuals and society. If we cast aside preconceived notions, we might be surprised by the successes in other countries.

"Of the people, by the people, for the people" - Abraham Lincoln

Chapter 6 – How to Murder Nonviolence

The "Us vs. Them" mentality is a constant threat; its destructive nature pervades both war and health care. There is a tendency to look at health care policy with the focus on the individual, without consideration for the needs of others. We must consider every side of an argument before we start making sacrifices.

Chapter 7 – Memorial Day

There is a lot of work that must be done in terms of foreign policy as well as health care reform. One is tempted to say that it is too big a task, that you and I are unqualified. We are a government of the people, by the people, and for the people, which means that it is our responsibility to get involved and use all of our talents, experiences, education and wisdom to make this country as healthy as possible. It will be worth the effort.

Chapter 8 – AmeriCAN or AmeriCAN'T

Democracy has been taken hostage by the media and our politicians creating a situation in which we are all so angry at each other that we've lost the ability to listen. This leaves a huge power vacuum in which our democracy has been hijacked. We no longer have a voice. Without a voice, we have no democracy for the people. It is time that we start talking to each other, debating substantive ideas with integrity, and figure out what we CAN, and must, do.

Chapter 9 – Burnt Out

Our medical malpractice system and its direct negative effects

"Of the people, by the people, for the people" - Abraham Lincoln

impact the quality (and cost) of care you receive. Most people think that malpractice only hurts the providers. While there is a very real price that providers pay during a malpractice lawsuit, patients often pay a heftier tax.

Chapter 10 – A Perfect Storm
What similarities do you share with my patient, Sam, who has a lifetime of poor daily health decisions? Sam is typical of millions of Americans whose lifestyles are bankrupting our medical system. Take a hard look in the mirror, question your role, and find out what you can do to help.

Chapter 11 – There Is No Enemy Here
Welcome to a day in the life of a doctor practicing in the USA, and what that means for your individual health and the care you get or do not get because of the medical system at play.

Chapter 12 – Putting Your Head in the Sand Only Makes It Harder to Breathe
What happens when nobody is willing to take responsibility for his/her part in the "health care" system? Lack of responsibility equals lack of accountability, which has led to our current unhealthful state of affairs.

Chapter 13 – The Doctor Will NOT See You Now
People often think that universal health care will mean a system like the Veterans Administration. Nothing could be further from the truth. This chapter will explore how France administers its system and how it can be a model for rebuilding ours.

"Of the people, by the people, for the people" - Abraham Lincoln

TENETS OF SOUND HEALTH CARE POLICY

The following will be expounded upon throughout the rest of the book. Upon these tenets, we will rebuild the "health care" system into something that is of the people, by the people and for the people!

Tenet 1: Optimal health frees people to secure, on their own terms, life, liberty, and the pursuit of happiness. Without health, our potential—both individually and societally—is blunted.

Tenet 2: Increasing the health of individuals will lead to a healthier, whole society.

Tenet 3: While an individual should not be required to make a specified set of healthful choices, each person should take responsibility for the sum of those choices; at the same time, the group should not be penalized for an individual's decision (such as rationing of care and/or resources).

Tenet 4: We need reasonable legal and administrative protections for our providers. We need to advocate for doctors so that they are supported in practicing essential medicine and not the defensive medicine that is also potentially invasive (and costly).

Tenet 5: Every piece of the health care system must be held to account, not just the provider.

Tenet 6: One should have abundant access to resources that promote wholesome choices.

"Of the people, by the people, for the people" - Abraham Lincoln

Tenet 7: Disease prevention is the highest priority.

Tenet 8: Advancements in health care knowledge and delivery should be encouraged, regardless of profitability.

Tenet 9: Health care needs to be affordable, accessible, and sustainable.

Tenet 10: Common sense, not overly obtrusive strategy, needs to rule.

Tenet 11: The system cannot tolerate fraud, waste, or the abuse of resources.

Tenet 12: Public health policy should encourage the entire population—blind to social influences while attentive to educational, regional, and cultural nuances.

Tenet 13: We should not sacrifice our rights to implement health care policy.

Tenet 14: Health care is not a partisan issue, and as such, partisan power-plays have no role in the discussion.

Tenet 15: Health care policy in the US needs to be constitutionally sound and supported by every branch of the government.

Tenet 16: Individuals, businesses, and the government should be able to anticipate their health care expenses year after year.

"Of the people, by the people, for the people" - Abraham Lincoln

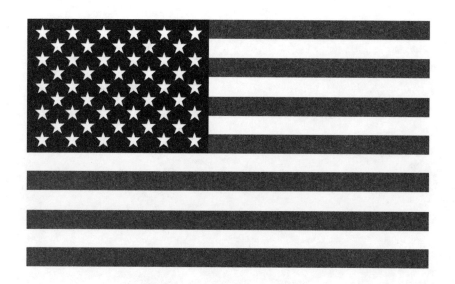

SECTION I

CHAPTER 1

LIGHT DISCIPLINE

"Winter is coming"
- **Lord Stark**

IT'S 102 DEGREES IN the middle of the night, and we are "nut to butt," a plane full of soldiers, sailors and Marines sitting on the floor of a C-130 in combat fatigues, helmets, and bulletproof vests, flying into Iraq. Now, "nut to butt" is precisely what you hope it isn't. While you might try to keep a little bit of space for yourself there are no seatbelts (just a strap across our collective nuts), and you soon realize that the closer you are to each other, the less you slide. Instead of ping-ponging around a plane that is in the process of a combat landing, we more or less move as a unit—which means more protection and less chance of getting your nuts into a more precarious position. They call loading a plane like this a "Floor Load" and you have about one or two feet between your nuts and another's butt = way too close for comfort.

An announcement comes over the loudspeaker: *"Strict light discipline in five minutes!"*

Light discipline isn't what you'd think. It means that we're not allowed to use any light source whatsoever. We cannot draw attention to ourselves as we do not want to be any more of a target than we already are. Think about a plane touching down. It effortlessly floats through the air—it's perfect target practice and the worst defensive position to be in, so we fade into the night sky with "strict light discipline." It works well enough, I suppose.

"Strict light discipline in four minutes."

It is in these moments when you start to think about your life, where you have been and where you want to go. Because it's better than being here. You think about your unfinished business, and you rewrite the lines you wish you had said.

My girlfriend at the time was beautiful, smart, and sexy in a librarian sort of way (she even wore librarian glasses). I wanted to marry her. My last memory of her was of kissing her goodbye at the airport. Her lenses were so foggy from tears that I couldn't see through them. I smiled, laughed, and told her, "It's only a couple of months," while wiping the tears from her cheeks.

Then, with a wisdom it took me years to understand, she said, "War was not made for people like you. I fear you will not come back to me."

Of course, I replied with something ridiculously manly and ignored it. Whatever she meant—that wasn't going to happen. As a military doctor, she had seen countless men and women go to war with an intact body and soul, and have only their bodies return. That wasn't going to be me; I would be the "unicorn" who came back stronger, wiser, smarter...

"Strict light discipline in three minutes."

I remember being thirsty. At the same time, I really needed

to urinate. This would not have played out well for the butt one foot in front of me.

"*Strict light discipline in two minutes!*"

The stench was obscene. Most of us had been traveling for five days straight. Layovers lasted one or two days, and each one was spent in a tent or on the tarmac or in an abandoned warehouse in Iraq or Kuwait. In the heat of the desert summer, temperatures reached 120 degrees before cooling to a balmy 95. We went to the bathroom in a Porta Potty. There were no showers available, no change of clothes that would stay clean beyond five minutes, and while we all looked tan, it wasn't due to sun exposure. It was a second skin—an opaque layer of grime. We were two minutes from danger, hours from home, and nauseated by our own stinking sweat.

SMELL OF DEATH

I didn't realize then how obscene we smelled. During combat, you experience fear, casualties, compromising situations, and a crisis of awakening that only comes after your soul has been murdered—but you have not accepted that truth yet. Even worse than this is the fact that you helped murder other souls, creating generational hatred.

At the end of the deployment on our way back to the USA, the Marines boarded the plane in alphabetical order, so I boarded first. We headed back home while hoping against all rationality that it would still recognize us, welcome us. When I approached the cabin door, the flight attendant—the first pretty woman I had seen in months—literally had to run to the bathroom to throw up. She was new, and her crew members had decided that the uninitiated would be the first one to greet the Marines. She wouldn't know that we would emit an odor so foul that no one would believe that it was produced by a live human. All the other flight attendants were already prepared with an enormous glob of Vicks VapoRub under their noses. They couldn't smell much. She was not so lucky. They were laughing while she cried uncontrollably. By that time, we understood how rank we were, and while this was a low point in my life, I couldn't see why she was bawling, as though she just witnessed something horrible. I wondered what type of animal I had become that could evoke this reaction. I was suddenly aware of the fact that I no longer belonged in civil society. It was not just an olfactory response to noxious stimuli— it was also the *cry of havoc* from an inexperienced soul locked in a cabin full of beasts, all rotting from the inside out. Nothing good was left inside of us. Her sobbing wasn't from grief or shock or sorrow. Her anguish was biblical in every sense. She had witnessed the living dead walk onto an airplane without the glimmer of life in their eyes. Our worst fear had come true. Instead of having enough decency to die and join our soul's fate in this war, we decided to return home in denial. And now, she was trapped in a metal shell with soulless Marines, hypervigilant to danger and numb to everything else, especially the stench of death.

LET THERE BE DARK

On my first flight into Iraq, the infectiously nauseating stench was about to boil over as the loudspeaker sputtered, *"Strict light discipline in one minute!"*

"Of the people, by the people, for the people" - Abraham Lincoln

Please. Nobody throw up. Please, please, nobody throw up.

"*Strict light discipline, strict light discipline, strict light discipline!!*" the voice echoed.

How one minute can take so long and then disappear in an instant is still a mystery to me.

Our imaginations can create fictions far worse than reality. Nothing happened for what seemed like a long time. Five minutes or more had passed in the dark, and I started to notice that the air was beginning to rot. I noticed that my legs were numb from sitting nut to butt. I saw the macabre madness that was about to play out.

This sucks.

But as soon as the miserable thoughts had surfaced, the world fell out from beneath us.

I should explain that combat landings are intense enough to rival any amusement park ride. Basically, the plane takes a nosedive, and you are descending so fast that you can hear the whistling of the plane barreling out of control, just like in the movies. Imagine the worst turbulence you've ever experienced, then triple it; plus, in this situation, you are sitting on the floor in pure darkness, except for a little green light poking your eyes from an instrument panel somewhere.

I had to wonder if this was purposeful...or if we were in trouble. While sliding around the floor, consummating the nut to butt experience with hundreds of others, we all were wondering who'd be the first to throw up—who would cause a chain reaction amongst the more sympathetic vomiters. I tasted salt in my mouth, thinking, *Please, if it happens, let me not be the first. Please, God—*

"Of the people, by the people, for the people" - Abraham Lincoln

"HOLY SHIT!"

In the last miserable second, the plane's nose juddered upward, causing all of us to fall back on one another. And about fifteen seconds later, we came to a skidding, Dukes-of-Hazard stop. That's when the cargo bay door catastrophically opened and a wall of sand tunneled into the plane. We had landed in what I would learn was a mild sandstorm; at the time, it felt anything but mild. A soldier stood outside with a red flashlight, screaming, "MOVE! MOVE! MOVE!" in a tone that left little doubt of the present threat.

Apparently, we had been shot at during the landing and mortars were currently being lobbed in our general direction. There really was no time to be scared or fearful. Honestly, I was just happy to have landed and to no longer be in an orgy of misery.

Welcome to Iraq.

War has a way of complicating these moments. In the process of being herded out of the plane, I had to gather the mission-essential equipment that I was responsible for—I was meeting my battalion and they needed a bunch of parachutes for the first "official" combat jump since Vietnam. This was a classified mission. No one could know what was hidden in those six bags so nobody but me knew their importance. Each one weighed about seventy pounds. Between the yells of "MOVE! MOVE! MOVE!" I picked up a bag and walked it ten feet. Then I had to go back to get the next one for two reasons: I couldn't leave a bag unattended, nor could I see the ground more than a few feet ahead of me and ten feet was certainly stretching it. I continued this process for what I guess was about 400 feet while mortars were landing somewhere on base. Since it was my first experience being shot at, I had no idea how close they were.

At that time, I was in ridiculous shape. I was 5'9", 175 lbs., 4% body fat, and I had more stamina than the average professional athlete. The bags were only about seventy pounds each. Yet, somehow the sandstorm seemed to make them immovable. I drowned in the sand. Absolutely everyone passed by me, running into the hangar and leaving me alone in the middle of nowhere. One at a time, I took the parachutes in the direction I hoped the hangar would be. This was my first lesson: I was not as valuable as a piece of equipment (since nobody knew how important the bags were, nobody stopped to help me), and no soldier was more important than the squabble of politicians (or we would not be here in the first place). At that point, I had more interest in finding the hangar and getting the sand out of my eyes, nose, mouth, ears, and lungs. There was no room for fear. Somehow, by the grace of God, I found the hangar, where everyone gawked at me, realizing that they could have helped instead of running for cover.

Once inside, I heard an exasperated voice calling, "Lieutenant Anderson!" The man had been trying to find me for the last fifteen minutes and had to be contemplating forming a search party. "You gotta go, sir! Your ride is leaving."

"I need some help with the bags."

"These fucking things got some weight to them! The hell you got in here, Doc—dead bodies?"

"Not sure. But they aren't moving on their own. Let's get 'em to the transport."

"Of the people, by the people, for the people" - Abraham Lincoln

Some Marines came over to help while I climbed into the helicopter. Thank God, the sandstorm was dying down. Throughout the flight we were greeted by locals as they fired small arms (pistols and rifles) at us. If it weren't for the fact that we were being hunted, then it would have been a beautiful sight. I could see the tracer rounds, streaking through the night sky—in our general direction—but I was grateful for the seat and because of a seatbelt, I felt secure (save for the unpleasant notion that a bullet might soon shoot through the floor and split me in half from the bottom up).

We had multiple stops scheduled that night. Since I was carrying mission-essential equipment, I was dropped off first. Being the naïve American, I had expected to be dropped off at another airport or hangar where I would be greeted by members of my battalion; then, they would take the parachutes off my hands and orient me to country. It seems like a silly thought now. That is the joy of being new to war and figuring out how things actually work.

I was dropped in a field, in the middle of nowhere, in the middle of the night, and while the sandstorm was done with, the winds were still raging. Sand peppered my face. "Walk that direction, Doc!" they said. And that was all. I had no idea if I were in hostile territory, or if this was Camp Fallujah, or if I had to walk a hundred feet or ten miles—

When I turned around to ask, the transport lifted off the ground, which only exacerbated the sand and wind taking their ounce of flesh. Chaos careened through my veins. I protected my face from the dirt, dust, and shit raping their way into every orifice of my body. That's when I felt a fear that permeated my soul.

"Of the people, by the people, for the people" - Abraham Lincoln

I wondered, *How fucking stupid can you be, Anderson?*

While trying to protect myself from the shitstorm of sand and debris, I completely lost track of my direction. I could not see more than thirty feet in front of me due to the wind and sand. There were no lights, no stars, no roads—nothing except fear and sand. I reached for my weapon on my right hip, crouched down to the earth, and freaked the fuck out.

Pure fear, fortunately, is felt by few. I had never been afraid before. Never. I believed that I had tasted it throughout my thirty years. I was wrong. All those other moments...jumping out of an airplane, the car crash, the fights, the anxiety about failing out of medical school, and the panic induced by a coding patient...those were uncomfortable situations—just nervousness, at its worst. Fear is a different animal altogether. Fear has flavor to it. A presence. It engulfs you, eats you without hesitation or remorse. Fear has no sound and its silence is deafening all at the same horrible moment. Fear consumes and fear destroys in a way that no amount of time, effort, or rebuilding can overcome. One cannot be made whole again. What's worse—it leaves a mark, and those acquainted with fear look different, move differently, and interact with everything in a way that is not complete. You know someone who has been eaten away by fear, and you distance yourself from them consciously and unconsciously because they're stuck in a reality that, instinctually, you absolutely want to avoid at all costs. Genuine fear is a world-altering event, and my girlfriend knew that once I tasted it, she would never see "me" again. I might come back physically but the man she fell in love with would die in Iraq. The queasy flight attendant sensed

"Of the people, by the people, for the people" - Abraham Lincoln

a slight portion of the fear I carried with me onto that plane heading back to civilization at the end of the deployment. She was simply too close, and it caused her to weep uncontrollably, while our stench made her vomit. In that sandstorm, fear seized me for the first time.

Crouching with my weapon holstered (but still in hand), I tried to calm down.

It's the reacting that gets you killed, I reminded myself.

After a while, I was able to relax enough to figure out the direction I needed to go, using my position and the location of the parachute bags thrown off the helicopter. But it was only a guess. So, bag by bag, I walked forward, hopefully in the direction of some friendly soul who could help.

I have no idea how long it took me to find a building. I also had no idea if I was headed in a straight line or if my movements were whimsically non-directional. It could have been five minutes or fifty because fear operates outside of time.

I found myself alone, repeating: *Don't turn anything on! Others might see the light!* Though I wanted to call out for help, fear silenced that, too: *You don't know who will answer!*

While carrying an extra 400+ pounds of secret-mission essential equipment, as well as my own gear, I was unable to see more than about thirty feet in any direction. Fear distorts everything that matters.

Where the fuck am I? My dreams make more sense than this shit!

Finally, after seeing a building with American military symbols on it, I recognized the USMC uniform on a Marine smoking outside. That was the sign that I was not in as much danger as I had imagined.

"Where am I?" I asked.

"Where the fuck you think you are? Disneyland?" he said with a smirk (until he glanced up and saw that I outranked him). "Sorry, sir." He mentioned his battalion, but I can't remember what he said. That wasn't my question.

"No, where are we? What base?"

"Camp Fallujah, sir," he replied, probably wondering what rock I crawled out from under.

"Where's First Reconnaissance Battalion?" I asked.

The irony here is that the First Reconnaissance Battalion (Recon BN) is full of a bunch of quasi-crazy, quasi-special forces Marines who should never be lost, and they would never ever admit to being anything other than cool, calm, and collected. And while I have no idea how I looked or smelled, I am sure as fuck certain that I was not managing my emotional state like an officer, a doctor, or even a sane human being should be.

"No, sir—I don't think Recon is on this base."

"You're fucking with me."

"No, sir. I've not seen those slimy motherfuckers on this base, but they tend to be sneaky as is."

"I need to speak to the officer on deck."

"Yes, sir."

It took about twenty minutes for this Marine's battalion to figure out that Recon BN was about three city blocks away, and when they finally got Recon BN on the radio, it was clear that they couldn't care less about their doctor's arrival.

"Of the people, by the people, for the people" - Abraham Lincoln

"How many packages does he have?" they wondered.

Ten minutes later, a jeep pulled up. We loaded the parachutes and drove to what would be my "home" for the next couple of months.

Now "home" connotes a place that is safe, comfortable, and somewhat stable. Camp Fallujah was no such place. Soon after, I was so worn out that I woke up from pseudo-sleep, needing to use the bathroom. I went outside and started to pee. Unfortunately, halfway through the stream, I put my penis back in my pants, still peeing. I was so worn out that I just didn't care, and I just kept going, walked back inside (pants completely soaked) and climbed back into my sleeping bag. This was no home.

The Marines snatched and opened the bags to inspect the parachutes, not introducing themselves, but finally, a master sergeant came and took me around the compound and showed me where I could sleep. Nobody cared that I was there. I had lain down for about an hour when fear woke me up with brutal pain, eviscerating my abdomen *From Left to Right*. It was pitch black in the room, and while I was sitting straight up, I didn't find light anywhere.

What the C-130 crew did not tell us was that once you enter Iraq, and once true fear has gripped you, the lights never turn back on. *Strict Light Discipline! Strict Light Discipline! Strict Light Discipline!* All the time. Darkness was our reality. Fear was consuming my bones. My humanity was choking to death. Welcome to the suck.

PERSPECTIVE

Looking back on that first night in war, it was all a metaphor for what was waiting for me as a civilian doctor with my own clinic, engaged in another kind of no less deadly conflict. But the difference is that, unlike the few who go to war, all of us—each of you—are going to one day be in your own version of that C-130 trying to survive the night. Only this time it will be a hospital bed and you will be reliant on the "system" to take care of you. But the "system," except hopefully for the medical personnel treating you, isn't designed to care about you. You are a number, an insurance claim, a prescription, a part of the corporate bottom line designed to make as much money off of you as possible. Just like in the C-130, there will be nobody who is capable of leading you through the experience and into safety because the "system" is so fractured that it is not up to the doctor to decide what procedure will be covered, what medication can be written, which rehab facility you can go to and for how long... All of these decisions are made by bean counters at the insurance companies whose job is NOT to get you better. Instead, they are trying to make more money for the shareholders. Much like me, blinded by a sandstorm, gripped with fear, and freaking the fuck out, so will you be one day, in a hospital room hoping against all hope that you are indeed in friendly territory even though absolutely everything else that surrounds you is witness to the contrary.

There are all kinds of suck in life, and everyone has had a life-altering situation, or they're living through it, or it's coming around. In the days and months of my first and second deployments to Fallujah, Iraq, I learned more about doctoring than I could have ever learned any other way. I experienced the fulfillment and the nightmare that come from helping people, Marines and Iraqi civilians alike, who needed and were grateful for

"Of the people, by the people, for the people" - Abraham Lincoln

the health care I could provide. And then I separated from the military, opened my own medical practice, and entered into a new kind conflict: that of trying to provide good medical care to patients in spite of the American medical system and the entitlement mentality that is infecting our culture.

Medicine is rife with suck. Inside out, and start to finish, medicine in the USA is the perfect engine to produce an epic amount of suck. Like the sins of the Catholic Church of antiquity, where knowledge was hoarded from the illiterate masses, modern medicine is also shrouded in jargon, enigmatic bureaucracy, devastating expense, fearmongering, restricted access to care, and defensive medicine (along with fraud, waste, and abuse by ALL parties involved—including you and me). When there is chaos, like sprinting from a C-130, it is everyone for him- or herself. There is no synergy of effort. Medicine in the USA is fractured. It is a shitstorm of epic proportions and it too is very much an "everyone for him- or herself" mindset.

While medical debt has been the leading cause of bankruptcy in the USA, access to care is atrocious and is rationed for the rich who have reliable health insurance (as inadequate health insurance decreases access to care = rationing). Deductibles are at an all-time high. Patients do not understand how medicine, medical insurance, or medical bureaucracy works. Physicians do not know how to properly care for patients when rules are in flux from government, insurance, and litigation; this translates to between 30 and 68% of physicians suffering from burn-out and physicians having the highest rates of suicide of any profession. The disease is a direct reflection of the environment that produced the symptoms. Defensive medicine is a failed system.

Each day I leave work with a mixture of feeling good that I helped others to the best of my ability, while feeling horrible about the absurd situations outside of my control that negatively affect my patients' lives. Some of these issues are self-induced by my patients. Some are resultant of the political climate, suffocating any prospect of sustainable policy. It does feel like I am still at war, surrounded by forces trying to harm and subdue. The house of medicine has been sliced in half, *From Left to Right*, evicting its miserable tenants, and plundering any hope of a healthy future filled with life, liberty, and the pursuit of happiness.

Welcome to the suck.

AFTER ACTION REVIEW:

- Do a Google Search for "Cost of medical care in the USA" and read a few articles to get acquainted with some of the financial issues facing health care. This book will be discussing many things but cost is certainly one of them, since there are simply not enough financial resources to go around or for the system to remain viable much longer.
- Do a Google Search for "How to stay healthy" and ask yourself how well you are taking care of yourself. Make a list below of what you have learned and what you will commit to in order to stay as healthy as possible for as long as possible.
- Ask not what your doctors can do for you; ask what you can do for yourself to never need a doctor.

"Of the people, by the people, for the people" - Abraham Lincoln

NOTES:

NOTES:

Chapter 2

From Left to Right

"When the rich wage war, it is the poor who die."
- Jean-Paul Sartre

MACHINE GUN FIRE ripped me open—*From Left to Right*. There were too many bullets. No way could I feel each wound. They blended together like a single strike of lightning. I was paralyzed by pain. It had taken root in me. The sorrow at what I had lost was so pure and consuming that I knew it belonged to everyone—it was the same sorrow all of mankind had experienced throughout the ages. At first, I only tasted trauma, oppressive and manipulative. The trauma murdered my soul, and then I felt sorrow and evil rip my guts out, *From Left to Right*. Most dreams are nonsensical, just a product of the imagination, and others are so grounded in reality that the mind remakes the moment, trying to master it. These nightmares become visceral. They have their own life.

When I shot up out of bed, I reached for my weapon and chambered a round, and then my eyes focused on my stomach. The pain was still there. My clothes were intact but soaked in sweat. There was no blood, no wound. I had never experienced anything that powerful while sleeping, and while I had no idea what it meant, I knew something was very wrong. It was adrenaline, fear, anxiety, empathy, and a horrible innate sense of self-preservation that were tearing me apart.

I was not equipped to process whatever happened to me, so "sleeping" was no longer an option. The nightmare continued to surface in flashes since the locals were still celebrating my arrival with sporadic mortar fire. Everyone expected me to pass out and be unaffected by the noise after spending a week traveling from Camp Pendleton, California to Fallujah, Iraq.

I put on my clothes and went to the communications room at Recon BN to ask if everything was okay. And while it should have been abundantly clear that nothing would ever be "okay" again, my goal was set—I could make others' lives better. I needed to bring some humanity, love, compassion, and talent to this war while trying first to do no harm.

The Marines probably thought I had suffered a head injury because I kept asking the one manning the radio, "Is everything okay???" They replied that everything was fine, but they had to be mistaken because my stomach felt like I was about to give birth to an alien; it clawed at my insides. Since I had only met a few people in the battalion at that point, several Marines were already questioning the sanity of their new battalion surgeon. By the grunting in response, evidently annoyed, I decided to go back to my room and try to sleep.

Nope. Not happening.

The adrenaline electrified my body, and my soul knew that this was not a coincidence. It meant something. I got up again

"Of the people, by the people, for the people" - Abraham Lincoln

and went back to the communications room, asking if everything was quiet.

They assured me it was.

I tried to familiarize myself with Recon BN and got ready for duty. I wasn't hungry, but I asked where breakfast was anyway, then headed in that direction. First, though, I checked in with Fallujah Surgical, the makeshift building where traumas were stabilized before the patients could be transferred to a higher echelon of care in Baghdad. The building wasn't suitable for livestock, let alone surgery.

There was blood on the floor of the central "stabilizing bay," which was a tight 400 square feet, plus a "Surgical Room" that was not fit to dissect worms. There was enough space for two patients in the stabilizing bay, which was filled with Iraqis and a mess of medical personnel tending them. I believe one was an adult who had been shot in the leg. The other was a child, about 11 years old, who had been nearly sliced in half at the waist by a Marine's machine-gun fire, *From Left to Right*. The child was writhing in pain as the medical assets were doing everything possible to save her life. In the chaos, she singled me out, and I looked at her. We both knew something about the other that we could not identify. Her initial resuscitation was almost over, and she was about to go into the Surgical Room for further stabilization. All I could do was stand there while a flurry of activity coursed around us. Her stomach was filleted open, and while mine was intact, we shared a moment that defies logic. She knew that she was about to die at the hands of the very people who wounded her.

"Of the people, by the people, for the people" - Abraham Lincoln

This is so wrong.

You're supposed to have decades left to live at eleven, not seconds.

Few things in life have hit me as hard as that moment, and the incident changed the course of both of our lives. She endured a living hell during the resuscitation, and then the recovery afterward. For me, the brutality and senselessness of that scene—the innocent little girl with her stomach ripped open, the medical personnel trying desperately to save her life in an inadequate medical facility—shook me to the core of my being. Even today that scene is vivid in my memory, and it has helped shape my conviction that medicine must be about providing the best possible medical care as and when needed, and not be driven by greed or hobbled by bureaucracy or manipulated by attorneys. That day in that makeshift surgical center, medical personnel did everything in their power to save that child and nothing else in the world mattered. Contrast that with American veterans who today, in the USA, cannot get adequate treatment for the physical, emotional, psychological, and spiritual wounds they suffered doing the job their country called on them to do, because of government red tape, frequently capricious decisions by non-medical clerks in insurance companies, or litigation that drives doctors to practice defensive medicine to try and protect themselves from lawsuits. In Iraq, in a war, in substandard conditions, an Iraqi child's life was all that mattered. There was a time in the USA when that was also the prime directive in medical care. That time has come and gone. We need to get it back.

My own dream-induced pain started at the same time this

child was mowed down. Then and there is when and where my faith in God died because God, the higher power, had allowed this unspeakable nightmare to happen. My hope for the future evaporated, all while helplessness chewed through my guts *From Left to Right.*

This was the same moment I realized that humanity is connected in a definitive, tangible, and spiritual way. A trigger-happy and scared Marine was likewise connected. He made an understandable mistake in the heat of the moment and accidentally destroyed this innocent little girl. His solitary action grew into horror, altering all of our lives. We are all intrinsically connected, and yet, we point weapons at each other, pulling triggers, and then we deal with a fragmented, amputated existence. War eviscerates us all.

*****

A signature facet of combat is understanding who the enemy is. But how do we define that? The enemy is not the person pointing a rifle at you—they are just a bystander who embodies an order. The enemy is not a weapon—guns are inanimate objects, perfectly good paperweights. The enemy is not another government because governments are only systems that bring order to a society that has either actively or passively adopted it. So what is the root of war? What allows this machine to tumble into different versions, and why is violence considered an answer to any problem?

I discovered the enemy in Iraq. It's sourced in the people who believe that their way of life, their philosophy, their religion,

"Of the people, by the people, for the people" - Abraham Lincoln

their epistemology is so fragile that it can't allow for a different point of view. The enemy is insecurity, ego, fear, isolationism, xenophobia, and power plays that benefit the "leaders," as opposed to the countless lives that will be destroyed by war, and the cultures that are torn in half. Whether we are talking about war or about health care, the enemy is the same: selfish ignorance, founded in an unwillingness to find common ground so the greater good can be achieved and so that blood is not needlessly spilt = first do no harm!

These adversarial views are enticing to the self-righteous. They believe that blood will get their point across, which is contradictory; after all, violence shows weakness. It is strength that finds common ground in the interests of progress, of peace, and the betterment of mankind. Still, few are willing to do the necessary hard work. It's easier to take young American men and women—often, they are struggling kids—and send them off to kill and be killed. It is easier to have a "health care" system that sort of takes care of the affluent and leaves those in the middle and lower socioeconomic classes to fend for themselves. Like most choices in life, there is what is right and what is easy, and the easy answer is almost always the wrong one.

The decision to go to war is easy, and it doesn't make heroes. The decision to deny health care to the masses is easy, and it doesn't create individual or societal health. Leaders who are compassionate, who can compromise, and are thoughtful in bringing health to the individual and the country are what is needed. You can be that leader!

Sadly, some wars are unavoidable. War was unavoidable to

stop Hitler from realizing his fascist dream; his ideologies were strangling Europe, and after Pearl Harbor, the Axis Powers (Germany, Japan, and Italy) could not be left unchallenged. Vietnam, Iraq, and Afghanistan are different. These wars are not within the dictates of what makes the USA, the USA—in my opinion. What's worse is that war's sacrifices are not felt by the ones in charge until the very end. Instead, especially in impoverished nations, it is often the disenfranchised, downtrodden, and oppressed people who were born without privilege who suffer; they execute the sins of leaders while fighting for the privileged (for those with better options). It's the same sin recurring throughout history: those who give the orders from on-high aren't the ones who carry out the atrocities. There is no sacrifice for the entitled—because they would *never* leave their sons or daughters in harm's way—and so their families remain unaffected by their decisions. What's worse, those in power often do not possess the wisdom and knowledge that come from personal experience of war to make such decisions. It is easy to send others off to fight, those who are strangers to you, especially when you have no personal experience in battle. You don't understand what you're asking them to do. But what of it? Soldiers, Airmen, Sailors, and Marines are unfortunately used as pawns, dying for someone else's gain.

And so is the same sin when it comes to health care. The rich have care and the poor do not. The rich make the laws because they, and their families, do not have to fight in the trenches of trying to survive a system which is so expensive, so cumbersome, and so shrouded in bureaucracy that it is simply out of

"Of the people, by the people, for the people" - Abraham Lincoln

reach for those who hold a less privileged socioeconomic status. It is the rich who often oppose any talk of universal health care because they are taken care of, and they think if others have their privilege that they will go without. Nothing could be further from the truth. Health care has to change.

*****

Weeks later, after a mass casualty, I went to the chow hall for a quick break from the chaos, and maybe get something to eat. Like locking myself in the bathroom at home to get some peace and quiet, sometimes the chow hall was the only place to decompress. Unfortunately, the metallic scent of blood lingered in my nose, plus the horrendous "food" was even less appealing than usual. But I was grateful to eat, surrounded by military—not wounded teenage Marines looking at me with eyes wide, brimming with fear, hoping that I could save them.

My sandwich consisted of two pieces of bread and an unidentifiable meat product. That was it. No lettuce, no tomato, no mayonnaise. They used to call military meals "Beans and Motherfucker" because you could find beans in every meal, but everything else was anyone's guess. Of course, there's always Tabasco sauce, which is so ubiquitous that we put it on everything. I guess even "Bread and Motherfucker" would taste okay with enough Tabasco.

The dining hall had big-screen TVs that displayed a recording of President Bush. He had apparently declared that we "won the war in Iraq." This was news to us. It was certainly news to the Marines in various stages of misery in Fallujah Surgical's stabilization bay. With the scent of young blood still in my nose, I—along with half of the chow hall—got up in silent solidarity. We left without eating. The hair on the back of my neck stood on end. No one looked up as we left the chow hall. No one wanted any support. No one wanted to be seen disrespecting our Commander-in-Chief. It was clear that we were disposable. Even though "inconsequential" lives were lost that day, according to our leader, we had "won the war!"

Only someone who has never had the personal experience of being to war would ever say that Iraq was "winnable." That would imply that it was worthwhile, and just like in *Ender's Game*, the ends justify the means. So we're good, right? Again, there is no such thing. But for me, for someone who was witnessing and suffering horrors that will be palpable for generations to come, I knew that there is no fucking way that Iraq could ever be won. *No fucking way*. War can serve justice, but when one side suffers even a single loss, there is no real winning. When murderers are put to death, we don't declare that we "won" the fight against them because their victims would disagree. President Bush's speech was met with absolute hopelessness, fueled by shame for volunteering to be a part of the war machine. I do not blame President Bush for what he said, as I understood his situation and the horrible choices he felt he had to make. But, that single press conference illuminated too much at once.

I remember the press conference when President Obama announced that the Affordable Care Act had just passed and I remember his face—he was not happy, not victorious, not hopeful.

"Of the people, by the people, for the people" - Abraham Lincoln

His face was that of someone who just lost a huge fight and I could not understand why he looked this way when his own historic bill had just been passed. But that is just it, President Obama's bill was not passed. The bill that had been passed was a lobbyist-destroyed-watered-down-and-mostly-ineffectual version that President Obama knew did not do enough. He knew he lost the battle and it was written all over his face. President Bush thought he won the war in Iraq and was mistaken. President Obama knew he lost the battle for health care reform and he was right.

Changing a system does not come easily. It is hard but enormously worthwhile work. It is the work that our politicians have not been willing to undertake as if their own personal life depended on it. Whether we are talking about foreign policy leading to war or public health policy leading to actual health care in this country, the time has come for us to elect the leaders, and for us to become the people, who will not surrender to warmongering or to lobbyists from enormous corporations who want to keep a fractured "health care" system broken instead of providing actual care to every citizen of this great country.

*****

I stood still, watching the corpsmen and doctors finish resuscitating the little girl for about twenty seconds before my instincts took over. I moved in to help. That one moment felt like a lifetime. We switched into the Surgical Room to complete the initial stabilization, and later that day, she was medevaced to Baghdad.

"Of the people, by the people, for the people" - Abraham Lincoln

I remember squatting in the hallway, staring at the blood on the floor from that little girl's stomach. But hers was not the only wound hemorrhaging in that room.

I walked to Recon BN to tell the Command what had happened (though I don't remember that clearly). They explained that another battalion had been ambushed the previous night and some of their Marines had been killed. They asked us, Recon BN, to accompany them back to the location to find the men responsible. When they kicked down the door to the house, it was very dark inside—one candle for such a big room. Everyone inside the home was startled, and when kids started to run, a Marine reacted prematurely, thinking they were enemy combatants. He killed two children, wounded an adult, and disemboweled a girl whose life was essentially over because in Iraq—even if we managed to keep her alive—she would be disowned by her family and within a few months she would die due to lack of resources and support. We had to try to save her, though the more "humane" thing to do might have been to let her pass without pain during the initial resuscitation. My soul still aches for everyone involved.

I asked the commanding officer how we were going to inform the little girl's parents of what had happened and how we could ensure that her parents could comfort her, so she would not be alone among the foreigners who shot her. To his credit, he realized the importance of going back to the house. Both sides had lost people in the incident, which means both parties are to blame, but none of that mattered. The only thing I cared about was this little girl—who was still in our control. I asked our

"Of the people, by the people, for the people" - Abraham Lincoln

commanding officer if I could go on this mission (because if the parents had any medical questions, it would be hard for the Marines to be accurate).

He agreed, saying, "Watch your six, Doc ("watch your six" means to "watch your back"). And remember what happened to the other battalion the night before."

I thanked him, realizing that this could leave my battalion without a doctor again, which meant it was the wrong call for the commanding officer to make. I also have enormous respect for his decision, because it was the right thing to do.

*****

While I had not met the commanding officer of Recon BN, we had spoken on a phone interview. During my time at U.S. Navy Dive School, I learned that Recon BN was the only assignment available with a combat deployment attached to it. My other classmates weren't interested in the position. I did not believe in violence as a matter of first recourse, so it was appealing to me to be deployed with some of the fiercest warriors on the planet, to work with them, because you can't be a genuine conditional pacifist unless you understand the risks, benefits and options bloodshed brings.

After the interview, Recon BN's commanding officer called his commanding general and asked for him to request me by name. This was highly unusual. The request was met with criticism from different sources, although among my classmates, this news was followed by a sigh of relief. They would not be headed to Iraq. To further secure the assignment I made sure that I graduated as the honorman (valedictorian) of the class so as to have my pick of assignments. Again, I chose Recon BN.

*****

Except for the commanding officer, Recon BN did not know any of this, but everyone in Recon BN had assumed I was the bottom of the barrel. After all, there were other assignments doctors who went to Dive School could choose from that were more glamorous and a whole lot easier. Nice, cushy positions—without all the dying—like I could have had with the pretty-boy-prima-donna Navy Seals. No doctor would choose to live the life of Marine Recon except for me. I wanted the most challenging and growth-oriented role possible for a doctor in the United States Armed Forces. And, there was nothing more hardcore for a doctor than battalion surgeon for Marine Recon. I asked for this experience. Hell, I even made sure to be at the top of my class (in case the interview with the commanding officer went poorly, I could still secure the position). All of this bad-assery amounted to nil. No amount of preparation, training, or mental fortitude can prepare you for the trauma of war. I arrived in Iraq weighing 175 lbs. with 4% body fat. A week later, I was 160 lbs. My mind, body, and spirit cannibalized themselves. It is funny how the perception of myself changed. I was this powerful, confident, vital, invincible doctor, and in seven days, I became a scrawny, scared, pissed-off and hypervigilant man-baby. And I would not change any of it, ever, because at the end of the day I brought light to the

"Of the people, by the people, for the people" - Abraham Lincoln

darkness of the Iraq War. While I was a part of the cog in the war machine, and because of this I am just as complicit as anyone else, I "first did no harm," did the best I could, and have lived another day to fight another fight—the fight to lead the USA to individual and societal health.

FIRST COMBAT MISSION

I had just volunteered to go on my first combat mission, and so the rest of the day was filled with fittings for the appropriate weapons, ammunition, and night-vision goggles. All of the equipment was in various stages of disrepair. The pistol that I had been issued looked like it had been dragged under a vehicle. I never even fired it prior to going on this combat mission and I had serious questions about whether a weapon in this state of disrepair would reliably fire. They found a Benelli 12-gauge shotgun and proceeded to instruct me on its basic operation. After four failed attempts to load the weapon, we recognized it for what it was: just a sandy paperweight. But that was all we had.

They shrugged, saying, "A little lube, Doc, and she will be good to go."

Then they dumped CLP synthetic gun oil down the barrel, pouring the full bottle in the chamber and trigger mechanism until it overflowed. I laughed, shaking my head as the Marine handed me a newly "functional" weapon that he had just turned into a newly repurposed shotgun/flamethrower, so I asked:

"What'll happen if I fire the weapon with this much oil in it?"

"I dunno. But best of luck!" he replied and walked away laughing.

"Of the people, by the people, for the people" - Abraham Lincoln

While the barrel was drying off, I tried on a pair of older monocular night-vision goggles with "Etch-a-Sketch" lenses. Like the shotgun, they worked, sort of. Maybe.

We left Camp Fallujah and drove to the house in the dead of night. The plan was for the Marines to secure the home, identify the parents, and bring me in to deliver the news. This plan seemed logical, except for the fact that I had not yet been initiated into the battalion. Had I met them in California, instead of Iraq, my initiation would have entailed rolling in poison oak, or a stint in the gas chamber without a functioning mask, or some other mundane, relatively harmless prank. In Iraq, though, there apparently were no benign initiations. The platoon decided that something more festive was in order.

The platoon commander, whom I outranked, yelled, "Dr. Anderson—out of the vehicle."

"The plan is to secure the building, first," I said.

He wasn't asking. "Out of the vehicle now, Dr. Anderson! Take your position at the end of the stack!"

You might wonder why he thought he could get away with that insubordination. The better question would be, "Why did I listen?" Because a seasoned, initiated officer would have smelled this nonsense a mile away and told the platoon commander to fuck off. I did not. I followed his directions, not noticing the smirk on his face.

A "stack" is what they call the procession of people who charge into a building after the door has been breached. People often assume that the first person through the door is the one in the most danger. That's not usually the case. After the door is

forced, the first couple in the stack infiltrate the room. The inhabitants of the breached room usually have no time to react; they are
just overwhelmed with shock and force. As long as the door is not
booby-trapped, and the people inside the house are not expecting you with rifles raised, then the first two in the stack should be
safe. The positions in the back of the stack are in more danger as
inhabitants in other rooms of the house will have time to rush in
right while you are entering the house. You don't want to be third,
definitely do not want to be fourth, and surely do not want to be in
the fifth position. I was placed at the end, the sixth position, with
absolutely NO FUCKING IDEA WHAT I WAS DOING.

It was pitch black out, no lights to guide us. My vision was
sketchy at best through the barely functioning night-vision goggles. The air was still. I did not know my heart could beat as fast
and as loud as it was. I waited for them to kick the door down.
I was still trying to get my night-vision goggles to work and not
having much luck; also, I had a dripping shotgun in one hand,
150 pounds of medical equipment and ammunition on my back,
and poor monocular (no depth perception) night-vision goggles crookedly strapped to my helmet, when a weapon peeked
around the corner of the house, just seven feet away.

F F F F F F F F F U U U U U U U U U C C C C C C C C K K K K K K
KK!!!!!!!!!!!!!!!!!!!!!!!!!!!!!!

An insurgent was flanking us, which meant there were insurgents inside the house expecting us. We had just a few seconds
until we were ambushed; we had a few seconds left to live.

*****

"Of the people, by the people, for the people" - Abraham Lincoln

I am a physician and a conditional pacifist—however, I was about to enter a violent house. Two days earlier, they killed Marines here. One day earlier, Marines came back and mortally wounded their children. I'm supposed to help put people back together, and I didn't come to Iraq to kill. The Marines have a suitable expression for this dilemma: "The best medicine is lead downfield." Meaning, point your weapon in the direction of the enemy, fire, and keep firing until they're all dead. Once you're safe, then you can try to save the ones still grumbling; then you get to "first do no harm."

I stopped fumbling with the night-vision goggles, raised the shotgun, took the safety off, and started to pull the trigger as the insurgent's body just cleared the corner of the building. As my finger was pulling tension, the stack kicked down the door, starting the assault. I was the meat of a shit sandwich. My mind felt like it was suffering a meltdown of nuclear proportions.

I went to Iraq because I was the best choice. I invited the adventure, the test to my beliefs with experience. I went to conquer fear—because I needed to know that, when stretched, I would be enough in and of myself. I went to Iraq to heal, not kill. I had something to prove to the world, but I also had a deep, affected desire to change what I could. I always ascribed to the notion that "If you do not see yourself as part of the problem, then you will never be a part of the solution." I knew that being a doctor in war was something that had to be done, and I would be the one to do it.

*****

"Of the people, by the people, for the people" - Abraham Lincoln

I had already made the decision to pull the trigger of the 12-gauge shotgun on another sentient human being, just seven feet away. I was at the end of a stack, charging a house filled (presumably) with enemy combatants. At seven feet, I would cut this human in half, coincidentally, *From Left to Right*.

As I engaged the trigger, I noticed a small 1cm-square infra-red patch on his arm— (see center photo section of this book to notice how small it is)

HOLY SHIT!!! It was not an enemy combatant. This is a fellow Marine! One of us! We were not walking into an ambush!

This is how they cleared a house. I would have known that if I had ever been involved in any sort of training on how to behave in combat, how to function within a stack, and all the other mundane fucking details of what the fuck we were doing there.

By the grace of God, I stopped squeezing the trigger and lowered the weapon in time; then a hand grabbed my shoulder to yank me into the house. All of this took place within about two seconds of time. It was chaos. The last Marine in the stack spun me around. Marines and Iraqis were yelling. Doors were being kicked down. Furniture had been flipped. Some people were tackled. Others were held at gunpoint while I was literally bouncing off the walls, people, and furniture—as I had no fucking idea where I was supposed to be or who I was supposed to be guarding, or neutralizing, or fucking playing cards with. It would have been comical, really, had I not just taken aim on a member of my own battalion, if it wasn't a terrifying situation, and had I not been there to tell a family the details about their

"Of the people, by the people, for the people" - Abraham Lincoln

dead and dying children. It was a fuck-stick of a situation and we were all getting raped.

*****

After the house was secured and everyone was gathered outside, the Iraqi interpreter asked who the parents of the children were. This simple question took about a minute of conversation between the Iraqi interpreter and members of the household. It made me nervous. A question followed by silence may have been expected, as everyone in the house just went through a traumatic experience, but the interpreter's question was met with an unnecessarily long back-and-forth dialogue. Something did not add up. When the interpreter told me that the parents were not there, I asked what that whole conversation was about. He told me that it was nothing, just that the parents weren't present. While I do not speak their language, the answer to a simple question should not have taken more than a few seconds to answer. They talked for a while, and I wondered what they were plotting.

When I told the interpreter to ask about the parents' location, another long conversation took place. Finally, he said they were in the house directly behind them. This was crushing news. With all the commotion, the neighbors knew precisely what was happening and would be prepared if we came knocking. This was anything but friendly territory. We had another problem, though. The only way to get to the house was on foot. It took us away from our Humvees that afforded weapon capabilities, quick transport options, and partial armor plating. Still, we had

"Of the people, by the people, for the people" - Abraham Lincoln

a job to do. And since it was more of a humanitarian than a combat mission, I was the one who opened my big mouth to the commanding officer. This was also my mission. The problem was that "doing the right thing" was inherently dangerous, which put more lives at risk.

We gathered those at the house and went to the neighbors'. Fortunately, they were outside waiting. I was instructed to guard all of the Iraqis while Marines secured the perimeter and interior of the house. Not really knowing what to do, I had the interpreter tell all fifteen to sit down. I held my shotgun and stood a good ten feet away from them because I was outnumbered. After five minutes, the Marines returned, laughing.

"Loosen up, Doc! You're scaring the locals." If only it had been funny.

I met the parents, but I don't remember much of the conversation. It was short. I paused to see if they had questions, and they asked how much we were going to pay them for their dead children, along with the wounded girl. The Marines expected this and handed me a stack of cash—about two years' salary for each child. The father counted the money, nodded, and walked away. That was it. Reparations were made in a single transaction with all the emotion of buying a gallon of milk.

The 11-year-old girl made it to Baghdad alive, and they were able to keep her alive until discharge. I completely lost track of her after that—there were no patient tracking systems that made their way back to Fallujah—so I asked our interpreter, who was an Iraqi citizen, what would happen to her. He told me that her family would not speak to her again, that she would be taken to a medical halfway house, that the facility would be incapable of meeting her needs, and that she would die soon after.

Is this the right thing? Wouldn't it be the civilized thing to just let her die at Fallujah Surgical? Of course, we can't ask these questions. We always have to try.

In the end, we prolonged her suffering, her sorrow, and let her die far away without her family. This is war. The next time you hear of men in combat, please remember this story because these stories are universal. The cause cannot "justify" countless horrors. If the fight does not outweigh the potential outcome, we need to find better ways of settling our differences.

I've questioned this encounter for years, and finally, after over a decade of trying to make sense of it, I have six working theories:

First, we are all more connected than we think. This is a profound statement and when we look at death, dying, and health care, we see that the more we do for the masses, the better our individual care will be. This plays out when you research health outcomes of countries that have universal health care vs what actually happens in the USA with our "health care." However, this requires that the masses hold themselves accountable or the system will not be sustainable or functional. All of us should do everything possible to take care of ourselves so that there are adequate resources for all.

Second, medicine is full of hard decisions; however, we have to live with those results, which can be fruitless (or potentially harmful). If we, as health care providers, start playing God, choosing who lives and who dies and how—without doing everything we can, when we can—then society will lose its soul.

"Of the people, by the people, for the people" - Abraham Lincoln

One of President Obama's advisors, Dr. Ezekiel Emanuel, wrote that the problem with medicine is that doctors try to do what is right for the patient, when they should make medical decisions while taking into account what resources are available and what is right for society. In other words, physicians should neglect to treat individuals whose care is too costly because society can't afford the bill. In fact, he has stated that when he turns 75 he will no longer get any medical care—no immunizations, no antibiotics for illnesses. He views that he has lived his purposeful life at that point and while he will not commit suicide, he will not consume any medical resources. I find his stance disgusting, misguided, dangerous, and in no way, shape, or form can we allow people like this to dictate health policy. The evils that will come from this type of thinking would be comparable to refusing to resuscitate that little 11-year-old girl because we had already decided that her life was not worth it. If we start making decisions that are above our collective pay grade as mortals, we will create new atrocities and the house of medicine will be in worse shape than it is now. Imagine if the story were different, that we allowed that little precious 11-year-old girl to die while we focused on the others deemed more valuable, or just went to lunch instead. What would your reaction be? As a society, we can't ration care, but as individuals, we must start taking care of ourselves so that the rationing of care is not the only option. Unfortunately, the current system of "health care" that we have in the USA is the worst kind of rationing and unless we do something about it now, it is only going to get worse until all of us are unable to get the care we need; much more on this later.

"Of the people, by the people, for the people" - Abraham Lincoln

Third, we have no control over the outcome when we "do the right thing." I'm sure Recon's commanding officer knew the danger we'd encounter when we went to find the father. He was wise enough to see that the mission's goal was worth risking the lives under his command. Fortunately, nobody was hurt, and it was the right decision—even if we had been attacked.

As our nation discusses health care policy, there will be some things that have to be done because they are right. Remember, there is always an easy answer, which is usually wrong. There are fundamental principles we must follow, like the rights to life, liberty, and the pursuit of happiness. Nonetheless, with all important principles, there are grey areas, places where nobody knows what the right thing actually is. We must have the moral courage to make decisions in these circumstances, knowing that there is no perfect way to move forward. This does not mean that people on both sides of the aisle, *From Left to Right,* fall on their swords in yet another epic power play that has nothing to do with what is right for our great country. It means that in order to craft comprehensive health care policy, we need to focus on the common goal: a healthy and just society of accountable citizens. Then, we can learn to compromise on the harder issues and meet our collective goals.

Leaders must be honest brokers of the grey, so that the greater good—*NOT* the greater ego—can flourish and create a sustainable plan where we all can thrive. The system currently in place is about to fracture because it can't handle the pressure of caring for an unhealthy population, each of whom is entitled to great care, even if they do not want to participate in it. When the entitled

"Of the people, by the people, for the people" - Abraham Lincoln

get sick due to poor choices, which is as immutable and as predictable as gravity, then they consume an enormous amount of resources (something that could have been avoided if they assumed personal responsibility and lived a healthful life). When a society is made up of individuals who are not willing to do their part to stay healthy, then no system is prepared to handle them.

Fourth, different cultures have different ways of dealing with life's challenges. In Iraq, the father knew there was nothing else he could do. He could not unmake the past, so he gathered all the resources he could, ensuring the rest of his family's survival. For generations, they have been so beaten down that he was not even able to grieve for his lost children. He did not have the luxury of mourning his children. Such luxuries are reserved for the privileged, for those who live in freedom and safety and abundance. In the USA, where health care policy is made by the privileged, the visions of politicians must be tempered with the perspective of those who do not have the same resources, mindset, perspective, or way of life. For a society to be just, ALL individuals need to subscribe to policies that work for everyone, while at the same time helping others to be their best selves. Policies must be for the people and by the people with no advantage for anyone to game the system.

Fifth, some life events will forever change you. There is nothing left to do but suck it up and move on because there is a full deployment left and a battalion of people depending on you. Process later. Help those who need your help now. Do the best you can and move on. No matter where you are in the world, this lesson is important: your needs do not matter in the moment.

"Of the people, by the people, for the people" - Abraham Lincoln

There is a greater mission at hand than wallowing in your own emotional swamp. Yes, it is hard to accept, and absolutely it is necessary. Growth without sacrifice is a unicorn experience— because it does not happen. We must be willing to endure hard times with matching consequences, so that the future is brighter than it would have been if we just floundered, disappointed in the difficulty of life. Push through. Have the integrity to realize that this is NOT about you, even though you are living through it. We have a responsibility to ourselves and to the following generations to push through, to do our best, to do the right thing, and make the world better.

And last, there is no communication without understanding. Just like when the interpreter was having long conversations over simple questions, how often do we ask simple questions about our "health care" and the answers we are given make absolutely no sense? We should have understandable answers to simple questions. If the system is so complex that not even the doctors who administer the system understand the system, how in the world is the system for the people and by the people?

I want to explore these six concepts further in the rest of the book as they relate to medical care in the USA, explaining these realities better than boring statistics and partisan nonsense. And if you ever wonder about my political affiliation, know that I have none. I am not a Republican and not a Democrat. **I'm an American and I am damn proud of it, of this country, and the future we will create for it.** Someday, if I am forced to choose a political party for the greater good, then I will do it reluctantly. Until then, I am an American who wants what is best for the

"Of the people, by the people, for the people" - Abraham Lincoln

USA, which means taking the challenging path, admitting personal liability and responsibility, and forging health care strategies that work for all willing to do their part.

Universal health care is often thought of as a leftward-leaning liberal platform, but in this book, I hope to show that it is also the fiscally, practically, and morally conservative approach that this country must adopt in order for us all to thrive. Some of you reading this last sentence will automatically want to object because of perhaps preconceived notions on what this would look like, what you fear you might personally lose if this happens, or because you belong to the rightward conservative platform and have been told that this is socialism. I promise you that it is not. I promise you that universal health care, if done properly, IS the fiscally conservative approach to health care and I also promise you, much like George Washington warned us in his farewell address, that if we are too enthusiastic about our political affiliations then "Rome too will fall." We need to eviscerate our preconceived constructs of what health care should and should not be, look at the facts, look at the successful and the unsuccessful models of health care across the planet, and then realize that we are all in this together, for the betterment of the country, not the betterment of our particular political party. *From Left to Right*, this book will take you from thinking that universal health care is a leftist pinko-commie construct to understanding the argument that it is actually a rightward-leaning conservative platform upon which we can all thrive. It's time we play "taps" on the "Universal Death Care" that we currently have, realize that universal health care is nonpartisan, and boldly lead us into a healthy future for us all, *From Left to Right*.

"Of the people, by the people, for the people" - Abraham Lincoln

AFTER ACTION REVIEW:

- Go through the six working theories above and thoughtfully consider your response to each one of them. As general constructs, do they make sense to you and how does our current "health care" system fit into each of them? Write your answers below as they will help guide you through the rest of the book. Most importantly, if you write what you think on each of them you will start to frame in your own mind solutions to make the system better. The more people we have thinking of the solutions, the sooner we will get the health care we deserve.

WORKING THEORIES:

1) We are all more connected than we think.

2) Medicine is full of hard decisions.

3) We have no control over the outcome when we "do the right thing."

4) Different cultures have different ways of dealing with life's challenges.

5) Some life events will change you forever.

6) There is no communication without understanding.

"Of the people, by the people, for the people" - Abraham Lincoln

NOTES:

NOTES:

CHAPTER 3

WHAT STARVES A MAN INTO THE FEAR OF LOVE AND SUCCESS?

"I've been asked a lot for my view on American health care.
Well, 'it would be a good idea,' to quote Gandhi."
-Paul Farmer

ROADSIDE BOMBS—or Improvised Explosive Devices (IEDs)—were one of the most devastating weapons exploited by insurgents in Iraq. Insurgents buried them in dirt roads and, when vehicles of sufficient weight rolled over them, they would detonate with viciously effective results. Sometimes, the IEDs were detonated remotely by scouts, just out of sight. Sometimes, IEDs were hidden in clumps of trash on the side of the road. Regardless, we were outmatched; even the armored Humvees were often no match for the power of these weapons. When one of Recon BN's convoys was hit, nobody was killed—however, one IED had turned the Humvee into an unrecognizable, tangled mass of metal. It looked like crumpled paper. When the injured Marines came back into Camp Fallujah, we had the added fun of removing shrapnel from the wounded. One of the Marines had an entry wound on his left temple, which tunneled between his skin and his skull before finding its home behind his ear. As hard as it is to believe, this was a minor injury. Most IEDs inflicted far more significant damage, death not the least of it.

In addition to the frequent maiming and death that resulted from an IED explosion, the fact that they were hidden from view until too late added to the frustration and fear they instilled. When we can't see something coming or we know that our lives can be upended by unseen forces over which we have little control, we can have two basic reactions: we can lash out in hopes of finding those responsible, or we can sort of resign ourselves to our fate, shrug, and keep putting one foot in front of the other as we live our lives. Drawing an analogy between the unseen IED that suddenly impacts our lives in war and the state of "health care" in the USA may seem farfetched, but consider this. "Health care" policy in the USA is so convoluted, so incoherent, so layered in bureaucracy that even for physicians it is confusing. And for most patients, trying to understand billing, and why they can't get the medicine their doctor says they need or why they can't get any care at all, is so maddening that many physicians and patients just shrug and resign themselves to "the system." At its best for those who have adequate medical coverage or are wealthy enough, the system works reasonably well and is the envy of much of the world. But, and this is important, for the millions who don't have adequate coverage or can't get in to see a provider and even for those who have coverage but also have excessively high deductibles or have a "pre-existing condition"— or live in a rural community with inadequate medical services or

"Of the people, by the people, for the people" - Abraham Lincoln

(shudder) are reliant on the Veterans Administration for medical care—what lies in wait, hidden behind actuarial tables and accountants and bureaucrats whose main goal is to save money or increase the corporate bottom line, or maybe worst of all, government functionaries who write policies and laws without one iota of experience in providing medical care and who might not even be subject to the medical policies they are forcing the rest of us to live by, "health care" in the USA is rife with medical policy and costly IEDs that can quite literally result in pain, suffering, financial ruin, and death. And the longer we wait to shine the light of truth, compassion, and sound financial management on this problem, the more certain it is that "death care" in the USA will come for each of us until the "system" finally implodes.

*****

Back in the USA, it was hard for my senses to adjust to the lack of danger. I tried to remember that I was relatively safe, that I didn't need to look for IEDs anymore. Instead, I saw threats everywhere. Trash day was particularly problematic because every fifty feet of every suburban neighborhood sidewalk was punctuated by trash containers (with the very unreal possibility of bombs tucked inside). Beautiful and sunny California featured safe, happy children, along with anxiety-riddled commutes to and from work. I didn't like going for walks because my mind would fabricate perils that were no more real than any of my suspicious thoughts. Months went by, and I stopped going on walks. I took long detours to avoid trash cans. I refused invita-

"Of the people, by the people, for the people" - Abraham Lincoln

tions to be social. Basically, I just stopped living. In all things, what you feed will grow. The cumulative result of sustained fear, uncertainty, and doubt isn't hard to imagine. Isolationism begets isolationism. And when you are not surrounded by people who bring you into their reality, you can get stuck in yours.

One day, after the second deployment, I decided I'd had enough of living in my head instead of living in the reality of beautiful SoCal. In the past, I had seen psychiatrists and psychologists, who never really provided any solace. They all said, in one form or another, "You are the most self-aware person I have ever counseled, so there is really nothing I can do for you." Once you are self-aware, all you need to do is follow your intuition, and time will eventually heal all wounds. Time puts everything in its proper place. Needless to say, this was discouraging since all I wanted was a drug that could help me process and stabilize; I needed something that would make everything comfortably numb because the spectrum of my emotions was limited to paranoia, confusion, and anger—none of which will yield a fulfilling life.

Instead of one pill, the psychiatrist told me that I should go on three times the maximum antidepressant dose to help me cope with what I had been through on my first deployment in addition to helping me through the upcoming deployment. So that's what I took until the truth of the situation hit me: I was not depressed. I had Post-Traumatic Stress Disorder (PTSD), which had me convinced that I would not be able to bring all my men back from the next deployment and that I wouldn't be coming home, either.

"Of the people, by the people, for the people" - Abraham Lincoln

Often in medicine, pills are not the answer...

After the second deployment to Iraq, while I felt desperate for peace, the military asked me to be the first doctor in USMC history to build up and run the medical assets for a new program: MARSOC (Marine Special Operations Command). For years, the USMC wanted to consider all Marines as "Special Operations" (because Marines really are a breed unto themselves), yet, it was well understood that USMC Recon Battalions were truly the Special Forces units within the USMC. This was never formal. So, across the U.S. military, we were always treated like the unworthy bastards of the Special Operations Commands. We did not receive the same quality gear, funding, consideration, or glory as the rest of the Special Operations community. We got the shit assignments, the shit accommodations, the shit everything that other Special Operations communities turned down for one reason or another. Typically, we were called for jobs that were just too dangerous, uncomfortable, or lacked the potential for acknowledgment. In fact, there were many missions that the Navy Seals turned down, and Recon took over, but with the formation of MARSOC we were no longer misfits. We would finally get support. It was a huge honor to be asked to set up the medical assets of MARSOC on the West Coast. I do not have the words to convey to you what an opportunity this was and what this job would have meant for the rest of my military career. This is how admirals are made. This is how the medical officers of the Marine Corps are made. It was a big deal. I felt awkward turning it down.

The detailer (the person in charge of my assignment) couldn't believe it either. He spent about fifteen minutes re-explaining the assignment while making sure that I understood what I was being offered, what it meant, what others thought of my service, what doors this would open, and the good I could do. It was discomfiting. I tried to tell him that I was not doing well and needed time to heal, but without a point of reference, he could not understand. Hell, *I* really could not understand it. It was time to let go and move on, or people would get hurt. I knew my mindset was shrinking, not expanding, and if you do not have the right mindset for this type of assignment, other people will suffer—that was something I could not allow. A few months later, I left Recon BN to transition out of the military and pursue a civilian dermatology residency program.

After turning down the MARSOC position, doing a military residency was also out of the question because, with my reputation as a Recon doctor, the military would likely not use me as a dermatologist when I was done. They would still use me as a combat doctor due to my record. I was told that I would likely spend 50% of my time at war and 50% of my time licking my wounds back in the USA. The path was clear. The military would use me until I got so burnt-out that I retired, separated from the military, or killed myself. As many physicians in the military find or create reasons to not deploy, and since I had proven myself to do well in combat—if I stayed in the military— I would not only do my share of deployments, but I would also do everyone else's. I had volunteered to go to Iraq because I was the best suited to go, and while I was proud that I ran towards the dangerous unknown, I also knew that time and perspective were needed before I would be any good to anyone. So, I left

Recon BN, went to another battalion, and started to transition out of the military. This was a good step. I needed separation. Still, it was also incredibly tough leaving the people I had bonded with, and even though we drove each other crazy, we shared a mutual respect.

If my last day at Recon BN was made into a movie, our conversation would have been interrupted with cutaways to memories of gunfire, weaving the story of Iraq into a collage of war-soaked realities. That day was full of taking boxes to my car, filling out the necessary paperwork to transfer to a new command, attending my last Recon BN command and staff meeting, and the funeral for a warrior. The fact that I did not self-destruct by the end of this day is one of many examples of God's grace.

Command and staff meetings at Recon BN are very similar to private business meetings with added formalities, traditions, and actual leadership. When the Commanding Officer (CO) enters the room, they begin with an "Attention on Deck." Nobody else sits down until appropriate deference is given to the position, power, and authority the CO holds. Then the CO conducts the meeting, allowing discussion to process relevant events. Unlike many of the civilian business meetings I've been a part of, command and staff meetings are regimented in nature, focused, and take only as long as it is necessary to hear all sides of the issue before determining a course of action. The CO behaves like a leader and, in my experience, could teach most civilian managers how to conduct a successful meeting.

That day, the CO announced that I was leaving the BN and introduced my replacement. Because this information was logistically necessary for all to know, this was customary, everyday behavior; what happened next was unusual. I never saw it before in the military, and I certainly never saw it at Recon BN—the CO went on in detail describing what I had done at Recon BN, for Recon BN, and how the success Recon BN had enjoyed in the last two deployments was partially due to my performance and leadership. One of the accomplishments that came straight from the hand of God was that every single person who came to me alive, stayed alive after my resuscitation. Everyone. Another gift was that I was able to bring every single sailor and Marine of Recon BN from two combat tours to Fallujah, Iraq, back to their children, spouse, parents, and friends. Every single one.

I was shocked, embarrassed, surprised, and quite frankly, I didn't think I deserved what the CO was saying. The CO started clapping and then the rest of the command element joined him. I hung my head in shame.

I do not deserve this.

Not here.

Not now.

Not for what I did.

Not for who I was.

Not for anything—

While they all applauded, I was writhing, agonizing in the attention because there was no perspective or healing at that point. I was ashamed I didn't do more and that I was complicit in every horrible atrocity that happened or will happen over there. After about fifteen seconds, they took pity and stopped clapping. They could see it was stinging. One of the company commanders wouldn't stop, though. He kept clapping and clapping until I looked up. When I finally did, he gave me a nod, which asked something to the effect of, "Do you understand the honor you were just given?"

I nodded back. Then, he stopped clapping. I am grateful he made me acknowledge what had happened because, in the ensuing years, I would go back to this moment to help pull me out of the self-loathing ridiculousness that framed my life. With over two years at Recon BN, I'd never seen anything like it. Nobody *ever* clapped for anyone. Nobody was given a send-off like this.

When it was through, we went to the funeral for one of our fallen. The day was sunny with a slight breeze and simply perfect, but I could not see or feel any of it. I had just been honored like I had never before seen and yet I felt like I just pulled off the biggest fraud in the history of military medicine. My soul, at this point in time, was rotten from the inside out and any light that was shone on it made it crawl into a dusty, dirty, and shameful corner, scurrying from the light like a cockroach. So, I scurried from the command and staff meeting, alone, to the funeral of a warrior, a colleague, a father, a good man, and a patient for whom I had a lot of respect.

The air of a military funeral is saturated with unrealized dreams, testosterone, dread, doubt, and sorrow. There's a bitterness in recognizing a comrade's death, in acknowledging the finality of death, in understanding that we failed him, and the truth that we, too, are breakable. While civilian services seem to be either celebratory or somber affairs, military funerals are a beast unto themselves.

"Of the people, by the people, for the people" - Abraham Lincoln

Sergeant B (SGT B) was a distinguished combat veteran of Recon BN who'd just returned from his third combat deployment. He was a tall, solid, and fun-loving fighter with poise—he made everyone around him better than they were. His confident and gentle spirit was always welcome, and I do not have a memory of him in which he did not greet me with a smile. He was a husband, a father, and an all-around good man—a good Marine. Like much of Recon BN, he was an adrenaline junkie, so when he got back from deployment, he sought after the high of feeling alive. His outlet was racing his motorcycle through the hills of Southern California, and on the last of these outings, he hit a patch of gravel on a steep turn and smashed into a concrete wall going 60 mph. He died instantly. This was his funeral.

At the end of the service, Gunny, the leader of SGT B's platoon, stood up and gave roll call for everyone in the platoon. One by one, Gunny called out everyone's name in the platoon to which, one by one, they yelled back, "HERE!" SGT B's was the last name to be called. Gunny called out his name and was met with silence. There was awkwardness in the waiting. Gunny called out "SGT B" a little louder. *Silence.* Louder still. *Silence.* Red-faced with rage, Gunny was yelling "SGT B!" at the top of his lungs. *Silence.* Now, Gunny was filled with so much anger and frustration that you could see spit flying from his mouth. He screamed as if trying a little harder would bring SGT B back to us. "**SGT B!**" *Silence.*

One last time, Gunny screamed as if he were summoning a furious battle cry, "**SGT B!!!**" Silence. We took our shots of adrenaline, letting it choke our hearts. Our fists clenched and

"Of the people, by the people, for the people" - Abraham Lincoln

then our souls shrank from the screams and the guilt. SGT B was gone forever. "Taps" started to play as SGT B's absence was recognized.

When I left the Recon compound that day, I felt hollow. I remember looking in the rearview mirror and thinking, *Holy shit. How much has happened in the last three years? It will take a lifetime to digest it all.*

I became a hermit after Recon BN. I worked, worked out, and then I spent a lot of time alone. I gave away everything I owned prior to the last deployment because I was sure I would die, and I didn't want to leave my parents with too much to clean up. Rebuilding was needed in all aspects. I started to buy furniture from Craigslist and refinished each piece. I also watched a ton of movies. I tended to be self-destructive because I felt empty inside and I wished that I had died in Iraq. For the last six months in the military, I did "Sick Call" for another battalion, biding my time.

Even though I grew up as a military brat, I had no idea of what life in the military was like, especially one serving with Marines. Though I had preconceived notions, some of them popularized by Hollywood which were far from authentic, nothing prepared me for war or the healing that was needed after war. During times of war, the military can't easily be defined or described adequately. Many people have tried to convey what it is like to be at war, but none of us can do it justice because war demands a certain mindset in order to survive its atrocities. You can't enter a battle peacefully, believing that everyone has your best interest at heart. That thinking will get you, and those around you, killed.

"Of the people, by the people, for the people" - Abraham Lincoln

You must embrace the warrior's sublime mentality. You need to be willing to do anything you are ordered to, without argument, or you might not live. And when you return to a peaceful USA, you need to cease that perception (which might now be defined as *criminal*). War also commands you to completely redefine yourself within a matter of a couple of days, conditioning your reactions to the environment. Switch mindsets/personas/identities when boots hit the ground. Switch again to assimilate back into a safe, civilized society/family/community. Switch again for the next deployment cycle. Switch again when you head home. Is it really that complicated? Isn't this why combat veterans have such a hard time adjusting? They bounce between realities—one in which most of their needs are met, and another where that is an impossibility. This bouncing is confusing and often happens in an instant when a loud noise, a sense of danger, or the feel of danger instantly brings our psyche back to war, even though everything else in the environment tells us we are safe in the USA spending time with our loved ones.

While I was hanging my head in shame during the applause at the command and staff meeting, I honestly had no idea why they were clapping. I did not know who I was. I didn't have an identity. I'd lost mine. Before the military, I knew who I was, what I stood for, my place in the world, my personal and vocational role in society; but after two tours in Iraq, I had lost everything that grounded me.

Am I dead inside?

Why is this happening?

Why can't I accept this?

"Of the people, by the people, for the people" - Abraham Lincoln

What do they see that I don't?

Do I believe in nonviolence still?

Am I a combat doctor who has participated in horrendous actions?

Or do I accept that, sometimes, the only cure is a bullet to the head?

Is there hope for any of us, for the military, for society, for the world?

What the fuck is wrong with me?

If you can't define who you are or what you believe in, then the world becomes a scary place. I was being congratulated for my successes at Recon BN, but I could not accept it. The other consequence of losing yourself is that you have nothing to offer to a romantic partner. All you can do is take, which leads to nothing healthy. As I was walking out of the funeral, and away from Recon BN, I felt a void inside of me. I had no idea how to fill it, so, over the next decade, I repeated the question: "What starves a man into the fear of love and success?" Finally, the answer came to me—a distorted identity is rooted in the belief that you are more important than you actually are and is founded on assumptions that have not been forged in fire.

I could not take the ovation from Recon BN because there was a part of me that thought I should have been able to stop the pain and suffering that I witnessed in Iraq. Subconsciously, I was so egotistical that I actually felt as though it was within my power to stop the whole war, and since I could not, I was complicit in all the bad that happened in Iraq. Now, these are not the thoughts of a sane person, but they had to be present

"Of the people, by the people, for the people" - Abraham Lincoln

for me to react the way I did. Even in a war zone, you need that sense of control. Still, the arrogance of thinking that I was solely responsible for everything starved my soul into thinking that anything I did, short of ending the war and all that went with it, was not enough. It's a ridiculous thought, rife with delusions of grandeur. I know that. Nonetheless, I believe that if you do not see yourself as part of the problem, you will never see yourself as part of the solution; and in my opinion, this universal truth and mindset has fueled significant, positive change in the world. For this mindset to be healthy, though, it has to be housed in souls that understand who they are, what they stand for, and where they will be effectual. They need to be grounded—and as I left the funeral, I knew that I was the exact opposite. For those of you who know someone who is living through PTSD, you'll recognize that these thoughts and feelings and reactions were classic manifestations of PTSD, and that the level of confusion and frustration and anger that PTSD brings is not something that can be magically cured with a pill. PTSD is systemic. It's pervasive. It's automatic. And it isn't something you just talk yourself out of or get over quickly. It took me years to learn to live with and then abate my PTSD. It takes daily concentration, honesty, and work—but it can be done, and when PTSD no longer has a grip on you, you become what you were created to be and are now coated in armor that has been singed to your flesh.

As I look back on the events that surrounded me on my last day as the First Reconnaissance Battalion Surgeon, I see the grace of God shining all around a hurting soul praying that the depravity I experienced over the past three years was simply not

"Of the people, by the people, for the people" - Abraham Lincoln

possible and that I was not complicit in it all. Humanity would never allow it. Prior to Iraq, I thought horror films were scary. After Iraq, horror films became cartoonish—more comedy than anything else. True horror is what one human can do to another human and then justify it based on force-fed propaganda. And they get away with it.

Plato said that in a just society, it must not be advantageous to do the wrong thing. I thought we had a just society in the USA. During the war, however, I saw real injustice. Before I went into medicine, I thought the medical system had ethics, but now I'm confident I was wrong. I no longer ask, "What starves a man into the fear of love and success?" because it's been solved. Now I ask, "What starves a society into the fear of abundance and collective health?"

To understand the state of "health care" in the USA and not just accept the politically expedient excuses and assurances that all is in order, we must first acknowledge some fundamental truths and ask some fundamental questions of ourselves and our country. The USA does not lack for resources or money, yet we hear the cry from politicians that we can't afford the cost of universal health care without raising taxes. Our medical training is, for the most part, excellent. Yet we are hemorrhaging physicians to the point that acute physician shortages are already upon us in certain specialties and geographic locations. The financial coffers of medical insurers and pharmaceutical companies are overflowing, yet citizens are forced to pay more each year for policies that frequently provide less service and/or have more restrictions than they had the year before. Americans spend a

"Of the people, by the people, for the people" - Abraham Lincoln

staggering amount of money on alcohol, drugs and cigarettes, yet many can't seem to be able to afford health insurance premiums. We as a country seem not to understand that we live in a time and in a country of great abundance and, insofar as "health care" is concerned, if people would take their own health seriously and not expect a magic pill or potion to undo years of unhealthful living, and if they would demand that the politicians they elect would actually think and act in the best interests of the country instead of pandering to whatever group or movement might get them reelected, then we could resurrect an American health care system truly focused on providing the best possible health care for those who need it. Until then, consider these facts taken from the Centers for Disease Control and the Center for Medicare and Medicaid Services:

- Currently in the USA, about 75% of men and 60% of women are overweight or obese! Yet, when we are polled, 89% of us say we are in good, very good, or excellent health. How can we be so delusional?
- At least 50% of all healthcare costs are directly attributable to four very preventable diseases that all stem from being overweight or obese!
- Currently, about 12% of Americans have diabetes and about 33% of Americans over 20 years of age have pre-diabetes. It is projected that by 2050, 33% of Americans will have diabetes!
- In 1960 the average cost of health care was $147 per capita. In 2017, the price was $10,739 per capita! However, in other developed countries that have universal health care, they usually spend less than half of what we spend on healthcare

"Of the people, by the people, for the people" - Abraham Lincoln

per capita AND, THEY HAVE BETTER HEALTH OUT-COMES THAN WE DO IN THE USA!!!

- In 1960 health care accounted for about 5% of Gross Domestic Product (GDP). Currently, health care accounts for about 18% of GDP and it is projected to get to 24% of GDP in the next five years if our current trends continue!
- Deductibles have more than doubled in the last ten years, which means that more and more money is needed by the patient to receive health care.
- Payroll taxes only cover about 50% of the costs of Medicare, and it is projected that Medicare will be bankrupt by 2030 if our current trends continue!

In the USA, we have a system of rationing health care based on socioeconomic status. If the above trends continue with exorbitant and exponential increased costs of health care, how long will it be before you, the reader, are no longer in the socio-economic class that gets "health care" in the USA? Those with wealth have abundant health care, along with the freedom to pursue life, liberty, and happiness. Those without, go without—in all aspects of their lives—because without your health, you have nothing.

In 2017, over 27 million non-elderly Americans went without insurance. Since the uninsured receive less preventative care, they also receive late diagnoses for disease, and, once diagnosed, these individuals receive less therapeutic care. Health insurance for this population would reduce death rates by 10-15%.[1] In

---

1 Claxton, Gary. (2019, August 21). "How does cost affect access to care?" Peterson-Kaiser Health System Tracker. Retrieved October 9, 2019, from healthsystemtracker.org/chart-collection/cost-affect-access-care/

"Of the people, by the people, for the people" - Abraham Lincoln

addition, better health would improve annual earnings 10-30% and reduce stress for almost 10% of the population. Moreover, those individuals in the lower socioeconomic status have twice the depression rates of the rest of society, and we all know how well we take care of ourselves when we are feeling depressed. In effect, the uninsured can't lift their eyes to the horizon because they're too busy looking at their feet.

I didn't know who I was after Iraq, and likewise, American "health care" has lost its identity. Health care is one of the largest industries and continues to grow much faster than inflation, which exacerbates the situation as society increasingly requires more and more services, at least 50% of which are due to chronic and completely preventable diseases that are horribly expensive. So many of us are so unhealthy that we simply can't afford the system we have now that is barely functioning, nor are we able to offer universal health care. Lack of universal health care creates a disparity among the classes, perpetuating a cycle of generational poverty, which begs a high price in both cash and cultural currency. This needs to stop. We have to start caring for ourselves enough to focus on our own personal and societal health instead of continuing down the path of self-destruction, holding on to a system that benefits nobody except the big corporations. What we have now is as insane as looking at trash bags in California and wondering if a bomb was underneath.

I had trouble accepting the acknowledgment of Recon BN because I knew that even though I tried the best I could, it was possible to do better and I was complicit in the war machine. It took years for me to process and reconcile the trauma of war,

"Of the people, by the people, for the people" - Abraham Lincoln

and similarly, it is hard for us to look at the current "health care" system and admit that it must shift its perspective. Many of the people reading this book will most likely have "health care" coverage. But if you are honest, I doubt many of you are happy with your "health care" and many of you are concerned for its future. Now is the time to consider what life would look like without coverage because if the above trends continue, you too will soon be without care.

- How would you feel about your choices on a daily basis?
- How would it impact your life if your basic health needs were not met?
- Would you still be able to earn what you do now? Would you have an education? Would you even take an interest in a book like this? Or, would all your mental energy be spent just trying to survive?
- How would your mindset be affected—in every aspect— and how would that perspective alter your past, present, and future?
- Would you feel like a second-class citizen simply because you could not afford to buy a "health care membership"— just like the other 90%?
- How would your health suffer? At what cost? What effect would this have now and in the future?

Humans are weird mammals, and we often revolt against things that we can't control or that we feel are unfair. Having limited access to health care can often produce paradoxical behavior in which one is forced to take more health risks. Like me, living the life of a hermit instead of being around people who

"Of the people, by the people, for the people" - Abraham Lincoln

could pull me out of the funk that I was in, many who do not have access to health care sink into poor habits. We can create disease. And since many illnesses develop due to years of bad choices, the consequences do not start to hit until we reach the Medicare age of 65 years old (especially considering that those over 55 years of age represent 29% of the population and consume about 56% of all health care costs). For those over 65 years of age, the government handles more than 80% of the bill. Improper health care for a lifetime leads to depression and hopelessness—a revolt against all things healthy.

By the way, the same logic applies to those with health care. Just as I suffered no real consequences for my self-destructive behavior, younger people won't see the implications for some time. So, they take their health for granted, and they put off taking care of themselves. These inattentions add up slowly, and then Medicare is tasked with delivering very expensive care. For me, fortunately, this period in my life lasted only a couple of years.

What will it be like for you when you need serious health care someday?

Do you fall into the 89% of us who think we are healthy, when in fact, we are overweight or obese?

These are the diseases that are a huge contributor to the chronic conditions bankrupting our "health care" system – and we seriously think we are healthy?

Regardless, from top to bottom, from individual habits to societal norms, we can all admit that the health care system needs an overhaul. We need to start asking tough questions. Why are

"Of the people, by the people, for the people" - Abraham Lincoln

we *Coping with the Enemy* instead of finding a system that will work for us all? What do we need to step away from? And what do we actively step towards in order to be individually and societally healthy? I stepped away from MARSOC and the honor and opportunity of a lifetime. There were enormous professional consequences to this decision, but in the end, my health was worth it.

What will you step away from, and more importantly, what will you step towards? We are *crying havoc* but what will we let slip: abundance and collective health or fear of love and success?

AFTER ACTION REVIEW:

- Ask yourself what hurt, what insecurity, what circumstance do you need to stop giving power to and what healthful habit, joy, or dream do you need to start focusing on in order to live an abundantly healthy life of your choosing? Write all of it down below. We all have crutches that we lean on from time to time. It is helpful to name them and understand them for what they are so that one day we can stand tall and proud on our own.

"Of the people, by the people, for the people" - Abraham Lincoln

NOTES:

NOTES:

CHAPTER 4

COPING WITH THE ENEMY

"We have met the enemy and he is us!"
-"Pogo" creator Walt Kelly's 20th-Century Parody of Perry's Quote

O
NE OF THE ISSUES concerning health care in the USA is that it is perceived (and sold) as an enormously complicated issue that defies solutions except to throw more money at it or make more rules to confuse everyone. So, Americans shrug, mumble some expletive about the government or insurance companies, and basically just stumble along trying to cope with their medical issues and the "system" that is supposedly there to help them. In fact, however, the American health care system and the issues with it and the solutions for it start with each one of us. But therein lies the rub. For each one of us to serve as a piece of the solution to our health care crises, we must first take responsibility for our own actions as well as for our own physical, mental, and emotional health. Unfortunately for a host of reasons, accepting responsibility and being held accountable for our actions is rapidly going out of fashion in our great country; it is much easier to blame someone or something

else for our troubles or for whatever we want but don't have. Getting out of this mindset, deciding to take responsibility and be accountable for our own health and then the health of our health care system, can be a difficult journey. But it is essential for our individual survival and for the survival of health care in the USA. In some ways, the discipline it takes to accomplish this mirrors the struggle faced by combat veterans as they attempt to re-integrate into "peacetime" society. For all the horror and fear combat causes, it also has a way of bringing essential things like survival and health care when you need it into very sharp if not painful focus. When fighting to regain the humanity that war shoves aside, the aftermath of war can serve as a reminder of both human frailty and human resiliency in the face of some-times daunting obstacles.

It is this frailty and resiliency that form the context of this chapter and this book. To illustrate this point, I offer my own journey from naïve doctor to hardened combat doctor to a dam-aged veteran trying to cope with emotional and mental pain in a "peacetime" environment. Eventually I fought for a truce be-tween the demons of war and the humanity that war stripped from me. The road to realization of each person's responsibility for his or her own health *and* to really look at, try to understand, and then exercise their power to force public officials to stop speechifying and start actually DOING SOMETHING INTEL-LIGENT about our health care system may not be as dramatic as a combat veteran's struggle to adjust to a civilian world, but there are enough similarities that the two constructs can co-exist and reinforce each other.

"Of the people, by the people, for the people" - Abraham Lincoln

The rest of this chapter, and much of this book, is an attempt to be vulnerable to the reader so that you can relate to me as someone who has struggled with a health issue and chooses to overcome this issue each and every day. It makes me stronger, wiser, and more in tune with my surroundings. But most importantly, it has given me my mission in life—to help you live your best life.

*****

If we weren't out on missions in Iraq, we were back at Camp Fallujah. There, we slept in trailers, went to the bathroom in different trailers, and showered in others. We went to our commands during the day and then walked back at night. Throughout the days and nights of my first deployment, we took constant rocket and mortar fire. The first month fried my nerves. When we heard the whine and felt the percussion of those first bomb blasts, we ran for cover under concrete bunkers that offered some protection but would not handle a direct hit or likely even a near miss. Afterward, we tried to collect ourselves and returned to business as usual, somewhat calmly. This was the first time I'd been shot at. It made the danger more palpable. Multiple times a day I had proof that another human was actively trying to kill me.

For the first month or so, we could not hide the anxiety conjured by this degree of hostility. After about six weeks of relentless attacks, we became complacent and stopped looking for shelter. We kept walking at an average pace while counting the foolish "newbies" running away. In honesty, we were jealous. They were

"Of the people, by the people, for the people" - Abraham Lincoln

not yet used to this newfound reality, so we were judgmental of how they were obviously shaken up by the rockets and mortars. The hardened among us actually started to take comfort in being shot at. If there was a morning in which we were not shot at we actually started to worry that something was wrong. The newbies were relieved. *Rookies.*

In combat, as in other extreme situations, we often compartmentalize facets of our identity to make it through the day. This is a necessary coping mechanism that we all do. Like a frog slowly being boiled alive, we often have no idea that we are being slowly killed while we compartmentalize and cope our way through it. The problem with this strategy is that we became indifferent to the trauma. For me, I became indifferent to the thought that I was being hunted; hell, I even missed it when they were not constantly trying to kill us. This mindset does nothing good for having a whole and healthy psyche. If we live this way for too long, compartmentalized as hardened *killers* (this is how Recon Marines greeted each other), the compassionate, more rational sides are actively and passively subdued. The little voice in the back of our head that reminds us what is right, urging us to try a nonviolent approach, fades and is silenced. This in turn blunts your emotions, for if you can't manage to evoke an emotion to a bomb exploding in your general vicinity, how the hell are you supposed to feel anything else? While we are stripped of our emotions, we're left with only the machinery needed to survive war. It's a painful process that leads to a fragmented reality of hypervigilance and flat-lined emotions.

To add kerosene to this fire, our military knows that we, as individuals, control very little. We are told where to go and what to do by our commanding officers, and violence is often the first and last solution. So, the softer sides of your persona are necessarily blunted; the aggressive sides are sharpened, and those experiences stay with you. They erase the good. It's a recipe for horrible, lifelong consequences facing combat veterans when they "return" home.

At the entrance of our Recon compound there was a sign with a Shakespeare quotation: "Cry 'Havoc!' and let slip the dogs of war." I thought this was badass when I first read it, but then I remembered what it really meant: it was a message that encouraged brutality; to unleash the war-sharpened; to let them destroy, pillage, or whatever else they wanted to do to the locals. It was not very badass at all but I am sure that nobody really thought about what this sign actually meant at Recon BN. They just thought it sounded cool. Regardless, Iraqis were killed, creating generational hatred, and Marines' souls were destroyed, creating a new reality in which "going home" would never really be possible again.

In all things—war, death, life, work, relationships, play— what you feed will grow. In a war zone, you're conditioned to be disciplined, obstinate, aggressive, and secluded in order to survive. The moment you try to de-compartmentalize is the same moment that demands that you reconcile ALL of what you did while deployed. It's hard to rediscover oneself when you know the government did not pull the trigger on another human. *You did.* And while it is convenient to play the blame game, attempting to erase the sin, any priest will tell you that there is no

"Of the people, by the people, for the people" - Abraham Lincoln

absolution until you accept responsibility. You need to confess, which means acknowledging that you were involved in some horrible situations.

The more that society lauds me as a hero, the more I revolt. When people use this bright and shiny word to describe me, I shrink away from the light because I know it is not a true descriptor. There's just too much cognitive dissonance between reality and society's labels (which tries to absolve society of its responsibility as well). I am not a hero. I was an instrument of war, and now, I need to work on reconciling all that was war and become a whole person again. Only something bigger—something extrinsic and separate—can grant the forgiveness I crave. If I try to forgive myself, then it falls flat. *How can I be clean when I got dirty on purpose?* With deliberate sin, there is no redemption unless it comes from a legitimate authority outside of ourselves.

For many people, religion is the place for answers to unanswerable questions or for forgiveness; others find comfort and solace in support groups or other forms of communion. There are, of course, other less healthy options. Unfortunately, I chose the less healthy options.

While they may say there are no atheists in foxholes, war can destroy faith, too. And though most people do "pray" when bullets are flying in their direction, that brand of faith isn't genuine; it is a duress-filled devotion that lasts a few minutes. I graduated from seminary prior to medical school, but even with this background I lost my faith in Iraq because God is just as complicit in the atrocities of war as I am. God allowed war to happen, just like I allowed war to happen in my own small little way. This is a

"Of the people, by the people, for the people" - Abraham Lincoln

hard pill to swallow as, at least for me, God has to be the one to give absolution.

If you don't believe in God, then I think the state of things is even worse because who now has the authority to forgive? The government said we were justified in everything we did, but a lot of what we did would be considered criminal back in the USA. If we actually believed that we were justified, then we would not have had all the problems that we did when we came back to the USA. So, who can forgive if you do not believe in God?

In order to move on, you need to understand that your actions in war are neither justified nor those of a monster. Next, you need to resign yourself to the fact that you have grown since war and if you had to do it all over again, you would do things very differently. Last, you have to look to the future and promise yourself that if the USA is ever thinking about going to war again, your perspective as a combat veteran is heard from the mountaintops.

*****

As extreme circumstances have the power to illuminate perspectives that would otherwise take lifetimes to discover, Iraq gave me more knowledge than I ever hoped to learn. The result has been both unwanted and enormously valuable. Over the past twelve years, my work as a civilian doctor has shown me that all of the things that happened in Iraq are the same things that occur in "normal" American life. There are obviously differences in degrees of intensity; nonetheless, civilians spend their lives

"Of the people, by the people, for the people" - Abraham Lincoln

similarly—subconsciously working out the same idiosyncrasies of the human condition as those of us who have been to war. The puzzle is the same, even though the insult is often lessened. Oftentimes, the combat veteran's only way to cope is to escape, but those who have not been to combat still have traumas that take a toll on the mind, body, and spirit. The consequences of these past hurts are often straightforward as solace is found in unhealthful behaviors that lead to disease (obesity; tobacco, drug and alcohol abuse); sometimes though, they are invisible. Aftereffects reverberate in the forms of depression, anxiety, self-destructive thoughts, and defeatist mindsets. Still, the human condition is ours to handle, in either healthful or unhealthful ways, and how we compartmentalize and cope will dictate our future. If we try to eat our emotions, then we become obese and/or diabetic, or we develop heart disease. Conversely, if we cope by thoughtfully evaluating our situation, fortifying our bodies with real food for optimal function, talking with trusted sources, and exercising, then we can overcome our trials; we can live our best lives as productive members of society (instead of a burden to ourselves, our families, and the government). One approach is selfish. It assumes that we have the right to destroy ourselves; this thinking takes away from others while those around us are disadvantaged and exploited. They suffer to make up for the cost. The second method is stable and mature, but it entails seeking out the help we need and doing our part, honoring ourselves and those around us. If we choose to be strong, we can contribute to the greater good instead of leeching off it.

"Of the people, by the people, for the people" - Abraham Lincoln

This week, I had a young man return to my clinic to determine if he had any additional skin cancers. His first skin cancer was diagnosed in his mid-twenties, and he was appropriately worried that sun damage would lead to multiple cancers in the future. After I conducted the exam, his mother wanted a word with me, so we walked back into the exam room. Once inside, she asked for my help because her son was too terrified to leave the house during the day. He wore tons of sunscreen, plus two or three sun shirts, and that prevented his skin from seeing any sun. All this left him miserable and concerned those around him. So, we spoke for a while, and he confided that he was prone to anxiety, and he was focusing all of it on one health issue, his skin cancers. In a sense, getting skin cancer was fortuitous in that it gave him a valid reason to be anxious. By the end of our conversation, he realized he needed help for his mental illness or he would spend the rest of his life looking to defend his actions with medical conditions instead of confronting the problem head-on and leading a life of his choosing. Hopefully, he will not choose to "cope" by going down the rabbit hole of creating external problems/diseases to avoid dealing with internal ones.

Another patient I had this week had the opposite approach. He had a growth on his skin that can be related to elevated levels of cholesterol. When I asked about this, he said that he had his blood drawn six months ago and his primary care physician (PCP) informed him that his cholesterol was too high. The PCP wanted to put him on a cholesterol-lowering medication immediately—no discussion, no list of options, no nutritional counseling. Nothing. When the patient did ask about his options, the doctor added that diet and exercise would also work. So, our patient took this advice to heart and started watching his portions, exercising moderately, and he lost twenty pounds in three months! When his cholesterol was rechecked, miraculously, it was well within normal limits. I would never fault the PCP for immediately resorting to medication because 99.9% of patients will not change their habits to improve their health. It's understandable. Eventually, providers burn out and the statistics right now in the USA are that 30-68% of physicians are burnt-out, depending on specialty! They're exhausted by an entire system that is poised to treat, and profit off of, disease instead of promoting and encouraging health; the entire system encourages us all to reach for the easiest answer: take a pill (did you know that in the USA, 48.4% of us have consumed at least one prescription medication in the last month!!!). However, this patient realized that he had been using food to cope with stress and decided to improve his habits—not just mask their effects.

In other words, we've all been to war. Each person struggles with something, and we each find a way to survive (by healthy or unhealthy means). Fortunately, eating one cheeseburger with fries and a milkshake doesn't sentence us to obesity. It won't inflict painful costs, but we will get what we consistently create. If we do choose to eat this way every day, then our selfish and myopic choices will add up. Doing a hundred pushups on one occasion doesn't make us strong. There's no room for change in that little time; however, a hundred pushups every day for months can have lasting benefits. Health or disease is a moment-by-moment decision that manifests our destiny. Positive, consistent

"Of the people, by the people, for the people" - Abraham Lincoln

decisions will help forge an amazingly healthy future in which we get to live out our dreams, feeling content with contributing more than we take. Bad daily habits lead to death, disease, and misery that echoes into the future. It produces a pathetic, parasitic life where we can never be fulfilled.

According to Cigna, 50% of adults have at least one very preventable chronic disease, and 86% of health care dollars in the US is spent treating chronic diseases.[2] In 2015, a Cigna study found that four PREVENTABLE diseases incurred roughly 50% of all health care costs (obesity, high cholesterol, high blood pressure, and increased blood sugar levels). This is a conservative estimate but it shows that at least half of all health care costs come from treating these four enormously preventable diseases. If people just cared enough to hold themselves personally responsible, if the USA could individually and collectively commit to becoming a healthier nation, we would have abundant resources to offer true health care without the rationing of disease care that we currently have. Instead, we are becoming machines producing ubiquitous disease. We simply can't keep up with the disease burden. But what if we were a society made up of citizens who took care of themselves? Then, every citizen could have abundant and affordable health care *if and only if* people assume accountability for preventing their own illnesses. It is worth noting that the healthiest 50% of the USA only consumes about 3% of all health care dollars! Imagine if we all were healthy—how many health care dollars do you think you would then consume? How high

---

2 David M Cordani, "Infographic: From Sick Care to Health Care," Report Prepared for by Cigna, https://www.cigna.com/about-us/healthcare-leadership/from-sick-care-to-health-care-infographic (accessed July 21, 2019)

"Of the people, by the people, for the people" - Abraham Lincoln

would your deductible now be? How much better would every aspect of your life be?

It is no wonder that our system is hemorrhaging. In America, about 75% of men and 60% of women are overweight or obese. Since obesity, high cholesterol, hypertension, and increased blood sugar are all intimately related to each other (the vast majority of these diseases are caused by poor diet and lack of exercise), it is easy to see the wastefulness. And no system can survive when the takers outnumber the givers. This must change.

Please, do not misunderstand...when I came back from Iraq, I was not living healthfully. I was barely functioning. I drank too much, engaged in unhealthy behaviors, and was stuck in an aggressive, confrontational mindset. When I was at a medical conference in New Orleans, dressed in a suit and tie, I walked the drug- and prostitute-stricken alleys, looking for a fight or to be mugged because I missed my war-induced adrenaline addiction. I picked bar fights with neo-Nazis in Detroit. I cried myself to sleep in a parking lot, mumbling, "Somebody, kill me." I was barely hanging on. I hurt myself on the outside so that I could be congruent with the pain in the remnants of my soul on the inside; but after a while, I realized I was not just hurting myself, I was hurting those around me. That was unacceptable. I decided to simply change.

It wasn't simple, however. The first step was asking why I engaged in reckless, unhealthy behavior. After that, I had to be mindful, stopping to examine each action I took, while I was taking it, and determining why I was doing it. I actually had to stop and ask whether or not it was logical to scope out the cars on the street—looking for bombs—as I passed through quiet, peaceful neighborhoods of the USA. Of course, it wasn't logical. I tried to overcompensate for the lack of control in Iraq by bringing the war mindset back to suburbia. I could control the shit out of this manufactured "reality" but the problem was that I was living in the past.

Next, I had to address everything I felt in Iraq and force myself to realize that where I was in the USA was not Iraq, that I was safe, that war was only in my mind, and that *only I could give it the power to continue.* This was uncomfortable because it meant going back to Iraq mentally each and every time I was triggered into a hypervigilant fight or flight response—something I never wanted to do—and then forcing myself to realize that whatever I was experiencing in the USA was different than what it meant if I experienced it in Iraq. At first, each one of these episodes took me about an hour to work through all the emotions and physical ramifications that were being experienced in a palpably real way. After five years, they only took a minute to get over. After ten years, it took a few seconds. Now, it is hardly a blip on the radar. But I had to care enough about those around me, as well as myself, to stop the nonsense, to stop feeding a war mindset and to start feeding the wonderfulness of the present reality that surrounded me.

So many of us are not willing to tackle our coping behavior and admit how it affects us, our loved ones, society. Instead, we let the destructive behavior craft our identity, like me walking alleys looking for a dangerous situation, because we have convinced ourselves that we have a *right* to feel this way. We believe

"Of the people, by the people, for the people" - Abraham Lincoln

we're justified in acting out due to our individual circumstances, whether it's dealing with war, skin cancer, or a divorce. In truth, there is no excuse because being selfish is rarely justified. Moreover, the more we engage in these behaviors, the more we become a diagnosis or a disease instead of being a fully functioning human.

For me, I focused on the true reason behind every destructive and unhealthy habit until I was no longer engaging in it—not because I am some master of self-control, but because I went through the complicated process of de-conditioning myself. I had to convince my mind that I was safe, not stuck in a war, and so the tools that I needed to survive a war zone were not required during times of peace. Things really turned positive when I had the emotional maturity to plan out how I would behave in new potentially threatening situations. I created answers to problems I had not yet met. And planning changed the game. No longer was I caught unaware. No longer would I be a victim of circumstance. I took control, and the more I chose to concentrate on constructive choices, the easier those choices were to make, and the more I became me instead of the label of PTSD. Still, the cornerstone of all of this growth was in asking for forgiveness from God and then forgiving myself for being complicit in everything that was war. You need to get to the root of the problem before a solid foundation can be laid for a recovery plan.

We have all been through our own wars, and every harmful habit we make is a mechanism—a gloss we use to conceal past traumas that we are still experiencing. We must be congruent with who we are inside and outside. Most men and women would

"Of the people, by the people, for the people" - Abraham Lincoln

avoid obesity if they tried to understand their emotional connection to food. There is no secret to the body's proper weight. Every library has books on the subject. A Google Search will result in hundreds of sites with useful information on how to eat healthfully, and even without a gym membership, many forms of exercise are free. We all know how to do better, but we must find the motivation to get there—without glossing over the facts we don't like. We are all at war with the past, present, and future. We all have traumas that we cope with via different mindsets and behaviors. In Fallujah, we got used to being shot at, so after a while, we did not find shelter even though we were facing imminent danger. Then, we laughed at the newbies. In America, we have grown accustomed to tiny dangers: eating poorly, not exercising, drinking too much. Even though we all know about the injuries we inflict on ourselves and our "health care" system, we do not care. We also get jealous. We often even judge and laugh at those who are healthy and make good choices. Now, we're good at compartmentalizing our lives, never acknowledging the exact reason for our unhealthful habits that are slowly boiling us alive. Few would choose to be obese and have health problems, but fewer still will do anything to stop it—apart from ordering diet soda with their super-sized fast-food extravaganza. And the reason why we don't make better choices, similar to the reason why I walked down the alleys of New Orleans, is that there is hidden pain in our pasts that we are "feeding" because we have never faced it and named it for what it actually is; we would rather have it exist and destroy us from the inside out than do the work that is needed to get past it and create a healthful future.

"Of the people, by the people, for the people" - Abraham Lincoln

I looked under cars for bombs in suburbia. While writing this sentence in a coffee shop, a customer ordered a 1,300-plus-calorie, caffeine- and sugar-infused Frappuccino with an extra shot of cream. My heart breaks for her while her heart is about to be poisoned. My choice to not walk over to the bunker in Fallujah and her decision to order such a ridiculous drink are the same sin; we are both in the same pot of water on the stove that is slowly getting hotter without our noticing the danger that we are in until it is too late.

Perhaps now is the time to declare that we are all fighting wars on different fronts, and maybe now is the time to start running for cover instead of ordering another cheeseburger with fries, diet soda, oh, and milkshake! Your life depends on this realization, as does the viability of health care in the USA.

Action Items for a Healthful Life:

- Step 1 – Recognize the specific behaviors and practices that are hurtful. Some of these might seem innocuous at first.
- Step 2 – Identify and understand the trauma that needs healing.
- Step 3 – Do the work to understand why you are doing what you are doing in each instance.
- Step 4 – Look critically at the situation, separating the present from the past.
- Step 5 – Care enough about yourself and those around you to choose health instead of death and disease.

I went to Iraq twice in a physical sense—and thousands of times, mentally, when I was safe back in the USA. I allowed war to "*Make A Hole!*" in my life and thereby gave war more power

"Of the people, by the people, for the people" - Abraham Lincoln

than it already had by feeding into that mindset when I was safe back in the USA. The day I woke up, the day I realized that I was perpetuating and feeding my own nightmare, is the day I started taking back control; I refused to lease any more space in my mind to war, to misery, to self-destruction. That day, I started living again as a human—not as a combat veteran with a PTSD diagnosis. That day, I took back control instead of being a victim. That day I started to once again be Reagan B. Anderson.

"Health care" in the USA is a vicious cycle of escalating costs, preventable diseases, and a system that feeds off of itself to promote disease instead of health. It is self-destructing and we have all seen and witnessed the warning signs for years. We have been coping with the enemy long enough as we have allowed it to *"Make A Hole!"* in every aspect of our lives, our society, and our economy. The time has come for us to take a hard look at what reality we are actually living in and decide what future we want for ourselves. Jump out of the hot water or keep wallowing in the pot, waiting to get boiled alive?

AFTER ACTION REVIEW:

- Much like the After Action Review of Chapter 3, spend some time outlining where you honestly are and where you want to be in your life and with your health. Then, spend some time asking what the ideal health care system would look like in the USA. Go ahead and dream. Put thoughts to paper and start thinking about how we can all start doing our part, in big and small ways, to accomplish this vision.

"Of the people, by the people, for the people" - Abraham Lincoln

NOTES:

NOTES:

CHAPTER 5

MAKE A HOLE!

"We owe our loyalty to each other and to our children's children, not to party politics."
-DaShanne Stokes

WAR IS BORING, like watching golf or bowling, 99% of the time. It is only punctuated 1% of the time by adrenaline-soaked chaos, and when boredom breeds complacency, you stop noticing the warning signs. The mind can only handle these severe fluctuations of reality so much until sensory overload sets in; then, it can no longer function properly. This happens right around six months of deployment and this is when the most casualties take place. Luckily, the Marines are smart. Our average deployment cycle was seven months. This meant that right around the time when the fog of war was so thick that we could no longer function well, we were sent home so that we could not function well amongst our families. At least back in the USA we just lost our loved ones instead of losing our lives in Iraq. First Reconnaissance Battalion after all was actually called First Divorce Battalion, because if you were not on your second or third spouse by 23 there was something wrong with you.

Six months into my second deployment to Fallujah, Iraq, the emotional shitshow consuming my psyche got worse and I was as burnt-out as one could be. The problem was that war was still happening. That meant casualties were pouring into Fallujah Surgical, and I was still one of the people who could fight back against the insanity and try to heal the wounded. Since I am very good at being a doctor in very stressful situations, I often found myself running to Fallujah Surgical when the all too frequent mass casualties arrived.

In order to competently and successfully run a mass casualty you have to take complete control of the situation, assess literally hundreds of pieces of information instantly, and make a myriad of flawless decisions over and over again even though you only have about 1% of the information/equipment/support needed. A good doctor uses common sense and instinct just as much as clinical skills and resources. A bad doctor fumbles in uncertainty and does not lead the medical team through the chaos. Even though my mind was clouded by the fog of war I only once let it affect being able to take care of a patient, a story we will explore in Chapter 6. What's worse, I had one year of experience outside of medical school, yet here I was—expected to handle things that usually required another five years of specialized trauma training along with a whole host of support and equipment that we simply did not have! My going into a mass casualty in a basically condemned building, with a fractured state of mind, with not nearly enough training to do what was required, with totally inadequate equipment to do this well, was insanity. Yet, this is what I did day in and day out for two combat deployments to Iraq when I was not outside the wire (outside Camp Fallujah and in unfriendly territory) and directly supporting the combat missions. Common sense and a sense of duty were the only things that carried me through.

When I heard that another battalion had been struck hard with upwards of ten casualties, I hung up the phone and ran down the hall, yelling, "*Make a hole!*" so I could run through the crowded hallway of Marines quickly. Seconds count during mass casualties and "*Make a hole!*" reduced the time needed to get to Fallujah Surgical by half a minute. While I appreciated the importance of getting to a mass casualty response immediately, Recon BN disagreed; in fact, I was counseled by the second in command who said that it is not appropriate for their doctor to run down the hall in an emergency. An ideal officer is perpetually "cool, calm, and collected," so when I ran down the hall shouting, "*Make a hole,*" it upset the Marines. I tried to explain that seconds count, and if he was the patient bleeding out on the table, would he prefer that I saunter in as traffic allowed or would he prefer that I "*make a hole*" and sprint? This was an unfair question because he was right. Being "cool, calm, and collected" in any circumstance is paramount, especially when a mass casualty is occurring.

Have you ever been in a situation in which, objectively, there is nothing wrong with the environment or the people present, but the hairs on the back of your neck stand up, your stomach clenches, and you feel that trouble is getting ready to pounce?

"Of the people, by the people, for the people" - Abraham Lincoln

During a mass casualty event, there always seemed to be a heaviness in the air that was in steep contrast to the sanity of practicing medicine in the USA. In war, the heaviness of trauma lingered in the ether and seemed to be fed by an evil presence. Half the time I did not know if I was fighting against a physical injury trying to kill the patient or a spiritual enemy that wanted to inflict as much pain as possible on everyone involved.

At the same time as feeling this evil presence, it also felt as if the souls I treated were uncontrollably rotting from the inside, while the traumatic damage was killing them from the outside. I wish I could give a better explanation, but we felt that there was another enemy in that room, even if we could not see it, touch it, name it, hear it, or even adequately describe it. But, it was very much present and palpable with every one of our senses.

At Fallujah Surgical I saw that the two most critically injured Marines were already being resuscitated. The trauma team did not need my help as they were about to pronounce them both dead; their injuries, and our capabilities in the middle of nowhere in a makeshift medical building with ancient equipment that barely functioned, were too severe to survive. So, I went to the next worst injured and got to work. This is how a mass casualty works; there are too many trauma victims and not enough medical personnel or resources. So, the ones who have little or no hope to survive are made comfortable; the ones who likely will be able to be saved are worked on until they either pull through or die; and the ones who are just in pain but do not likely have life-threatening injuries wait. Hundreds of snap judgments are happening and all involve hope that we are passing

"Of the people, by the people, for the people" - Abraham Lincoln

judgment wisely, because the decisions we make have life-or-death implications.

After responding to many mass casualty events, I typically knew who was going to pull through, and though it's hard when resources are limited, you must move on to the next viable patient so that you can save as many as possible. Again, by the grace of God, anyone I ever worked on lived. But that does not mean that death and dying were not surrounding us all during the resuscitations. Tragically, there would be no saving the two most injured Marines who were about to die.

When you are confronted with a young man, someone too young to legally consume alcohol, whom you need to let die so that others can hopefully be saved, your soul hemorrhages and a part of you dies with him. These are wounds that never heal and never should be allowed to heal. Even without blood on my hands, even though I was not part of these two trauma resuscitations, the absolute rage inside of me hit a fever pitch.

I went to the next wounded Marine, who had multiple non-life-threatening injuries to his head and neck, torso, and arms. The right side of his face had been ripped apart by a shrapnel blast. As my gaze traveled from his nose to his ear, the wounds got exponentially worse. He was missing the lower half of his right ear, and what remained of his right eye was in its socket—but it was destroyed. His left eye would likely never function again either. I saw his eye protection was still fastened to his shirt (had he worn it, he would have saved his eyes and the damage to his face would have been greatly mitigated).

Full stop

"Of the people, by the people, for the people" - Abraham Lincoln

Something just happened and I need to explain it because I need you, the reader, to understand that while the words on the page are a sterile black and white, the emotion behind them is very painful. These stories are hard to write, but I hope they give life to the book and help you frame war and health care in a very real way that eventually inspires you to get involved and help change the system for the betterment of all of us.

I typed this story in front of my wife. She was working on the opposite side of the table and looked up at me, laughing and saying, "You all right?" as I buried my face in my hands, my body shook, and since she had never seen me cry before, she thought I was laughing. The tears felt shameful, awkward. When she realized I was crying, she came over and held me, and while this was a beautiful gesture from an amazingly wonderful woman, it felt foreign to be comforted...or to need comforting.

In the last fifteen years, since my first deployment, this is the fourth time I have cried. But why? How many of my family members have died? How many relationships have ended? How many Hallmark commercials have I watched? Yet, none of those triggered this much of an emotional response as typing this chapter.

For people who have PTSD, our memories are skewed, not accurate, and not really memories. People with PTSD do not really remember the traumatic events because our minds are still not able to fully process what happened, what it means, and then to compartmentalize it appropriately in the part of our brains that remembers. Instead, people with PTSD relive the experience over and over again in a sensory fashion. It is our brain's attempt to try to reconcile the trauma, since it does not make

"Of the people, by the people, for the people" - Abraham Lincoln

sense, invoke the entire body and all of the senses so that we can relive the trauma and hopefully this time put it in its proper place. I did not cry in Iraq over this story because my emotional state would not allow me to cry. Now that I have distance and health, my brain is no longer reliving the stories with fits of anger; it is starting to remember them with emotional catharsis, because now I can process them. However, after this much time I am again not sure how accurate the details are after having relived the memories so many times. One thing is for sure though, these are stories that are worthy of shedding tears.

As I type this I am reminded of the four different times I cried, as all of them are wrapped around the trauma of Iraq on a young man's psyche, the guilt of being part of the war machine, and the sorrow of knowing that we created generational hatred. It has been thirteen years since Iraq and yet it still has a hold on me. And this is a very, very good thing because it allows me a wisdom that will help lead this generation and the next into a more peaceful future. If you have not felt the carnage of war into the deepest part of your being then I am not sure you are qualified to make the decision to send our brothers and sisters in the military off to fight. The veterans of our great country have a perspective that must be heard and felt in every corner of our government so that if we do decide to go to war again, everyone involved knows exactly what that means, personally and viscerally. We must "be the change you wish to see in the world" (Mahatma Gandhi), regardless of the cost.

*****

"Of the people, by the people, for the people" - Abraham Lincoln

I looked at the Marine's face, and it enraged me to see such useless damage. Unmitigated. Preventable. Needlessly blind at 19. Even though this 19-year-old was suffering, couldn't see out of his right eye, barely out of his left eye, and couldn't hear very well, all he wanted to know was if the other Marines, his "brothers and sisters" were okay. He kept asking, and I kept lying.

"They will be okay!" I said, while triaging his wounds and treating the most serious ones first. I had to lie for if I told the truth, that his brothers-in-arms were dying, his resuscitation would have gotten even more out of control than it was due to the circumstances.

He was given narcotics during the resuscitation, but they didn't seem to touch his pain. His pulse elevated. He was sweating, breathing hard, writhing, and though he was now stabilized, he was still in considerable pain. Eventually we were able to tend to all of his wounds, stabilize him for transport, and get his physical pain under control. Now that his life was not in jeopardy, I told him.

His brothers-in-arms had died during his resuscitation. He looked at me with his one barely functional eye, laid his head on the pillow, and made a hole for his soul to writhe in. He had known the whole time that his fellow Marines in triage were perishing, and he felt that he was supposed to be dying with them. The sadness he felt was a jumble of remorse, rage, abandonment, and despair. Not a part of him cared about his own injuries. (The bond/integrity/faithfulness of our military to each other is so strong that we care more about each other than we ever will for ourselves. Even in these horrible situations, there is amazing grace

"Of the people, by the people, for the people" - Abraham Lincoln

that fills the halls, that is if you take the time to see it along-side the carnage.) We had a rapport with each other that went beyond our military heritage, as both of us were hollow with rage and remorse. We put him on transport to Baghdad. I only hope that what was left of his soul was able to leave that gurney along with his body and live a better life with Iraq well behind him.

Afterward, I went back to Recon BN to attend a command and staff meeting where we were welcoming and educating the Recon Marines replacing us. Each of us gave them the list of threats and tools needed to be successful in the area of operation. When my turn came, nobody listened to the medical briefing. Having just come from a mass casualty, and still having that Marine's blood on my clothes, I snapped. I jumped up on the table and continued my presentation in a not-so-professional manner. I predicted the casualties they would have if they did not take medical considerations seriously. I told them that I had just treated Marines in a mass casualty event, and how one 19-year-old had sustained completely preventable injuries that likely resulted in blindness because he wasn't wearing the ballistic glasses that were coolly hanging off of his shirt instead of on his face. I explained that in another instance, a Marine was driving recklessly and caused a wreck, which killed everyone in the vehicle. In five minutes, I vomited knowledge on them that, if they listened, would ensure that they had a deployment with fewer needless casualties. They did not listen to my public health messages. They did not listen because they were not in a mindset to listen, because who cares about medical concerns when there

"Of the people, by the people, for the people" - Abraham Lincoln

are bullets and bombs to heed. Simply put, they did not care about their health. Sound familiar? Sound like the frog getting boiled alive? Same same.

I was trying my best to give them active policies to follow and if they did follow them, lives and limbs would be saved. Even with my uniform having fresh Marine blood on it from a mass casualty thirty minutes prior, even with the well-known and respected reputation I had earned, even with me jumping on the table, foaming at the mouth and giving them active strategies to follow from a hardened combat veteran, even with— They didn't listen. They ignored my advice and because of it, people were needlessly hurt during their deployment. No surprise really when I think about it because this is just like it is in the USA. We don't listen to our experts. We don't eat well. We don't exercise as we should. We *don't*. We also don't research topics like universal health care for ourselves to see how other countries do it and what the lessons learned are so that we do not make the same mistakes. We just instinctually say that we either like the idea or hate the idea based on a political ideology. Just as in that command and staff meeting in Iraq, it seems as if no matter what the experts say, how we say it, what evidence we have when we say it, people are unwilling to listen to us and become educated on their own health, on our country's health, how health is done in other countries, what works and what does not work in other countries. We just keep dogmatically insisting that whatever we believe on the subject is ignorantly and categorically correct. This has to stop. I have no problem with someone disagreeing with me on public or personal health as long as they are informed. Unfortunately, few have taken the time to see if their religiously held beliefs on our "health care" system can be substantiated. When we have a populace that is more interested in posting what cereal they ate this morning on social media than they are in being actively involved in their own health, the intellectually robust vacuum that results unfortunately puts all the power into the hands of the politicians. Scary indeed!

One of the problems with war is that the people who make the decision to fight are rarely, if ever, the ones who have fought or will fight, and so they really have no idea what consequences will result from their vote. One of the problems with public health policy in the USA is that the people who write the laws tend to be people who are fairly affluent, well educated, and have never actually been a part of delivering health care to a patient. Therefore, their view is skewed and their experience is limited, so they tend to make laws that will work for them because that is all they know. The problem is that while the laws they devise, usually "active public health policies," might work for them, there is a whole segment of the population for whom the laws do not work at all since they need more "passive" public health policies.

Active public health policies are things like Health Savings Accounts (HSAs) in which you deposit tax-deductible money for health care expenses. Active measures require action on our part, and they are good policies for those who have the resources to know about the policy and are willing and able to follow them. The problem is that often, active public health policies only work for the relatively educated and affluent: citizens with resources.

"Of the people, by the people, for the people" - Abraham Lincoln

Passive public health policies do not require anyone to do anything out of the norm to get the benefit. Fluoride in the water is an example of a passive public health policy because people do what they normally do anyway, drink water, and then we all profit from the benefits.

Historically, Congress tends to pass laws that require active participation in the measure for individual and societal benefit, because these measures are simpler and because everyone in Congress is reasonably educated and affluent, so they consider policies and laws that help voters in similar situations; this is what they know. The problem with this is that you don't know what you don't know, and if you have never grown up in poverty or with personal health challenges of a serious nature, it is tough to relate to people who do. Still, everyone needs health care as a starting point. For without health, you really have nothing.

An unintended consequence of many active public health policies is that they create a deeper divide between the "haves" and the "have-nots." There are policies that the privileged take advantage of because of two reasons: 1) they know about them, and 2) their basic needs have been met (housing, food, security, safety), allowing this population the luxury of investing in things like HSAs. But as for the less affluent who are just trying to survive—they do not have the luxury of putting money away for potential future medical expenses. Remember the story about the man who took the money we handed him for reparations for his children being killed? He did not have the luxury to mourn. He just needed to survive and help the rest of his family survive. Unfortunately, when your basic human needs are not

"Of the people, by the people, for the people" - Abraham Lincoln

met, survival mode takes over and there is no room for anything active. You are just trying to survive, and when you are just trying to survive there is little left to pay attention to with regard to your health. Active policies simply do not work for people in survival mode.

Unfortunately, this gives the "haves" yet another unfair advantage over the "have-nots," who often 1) do not know about the programs in the first place, and 2) struggle to meet basic human needs to survive on a daily basis. Their concerns often focus on food, shelter, and security—they do not have time for lofty public health measures that might increase their standard of living or health. While these measures are useful for those who can take advantage of them, they also hurt the underprivileged, making them more of an outsider to the club of the healthy. It is a vicious circle.

To give an example further clarifying the difference between active and passive public health policies, let's look at the resuscitation of the Marine earlier in the chapter. When I was working on him, I was essentially employing a passive policy in that the resuscitation did not require him to do anything but listen (which he was already doing). An active policy would have expected him to participate in his care; at that moment, the only thing I needed him to do was to remain still and allow us to stabilize him for transport to Baghdad where more medical resources were available. Had I asked him to be involved in his own health care at that moment, like put in a catheter, insert his own IV, or stop his own bleeding wounds while I went to go get a coffee, then we would be justifiably horrified and ask what in

"Of the people, by the people, for the people" - Abraham Lincoln

the world was happening. The Marine was not in a space to do these things for himself by any stretch of the imagination—he had likely never been trained to put in an IV, could not see.

Similarly, many of the less affluent are in the same position in the USA. They do not have the knowledge or resources needed to take advantage of the active public health policies that are available. Asking them to enroll in an HSA account, for example, is just as ludicrous as asking the Marine to put in his own IV. Yet, we tend to shake our heads when the people do not engage in practical health programs! From their perspective, however, they are only getting by, trying to feed, clothe, and protect their families. They don't have the luxury of taking advantage of the active programs because their basic human needs are nowhere close to being met.

After war, my mindset was wrecked. If you came to me explaining how my behaviors alienated my loved ones, making them uncomfortable, and rendering me paranoid and aggressive, then I would have callously turned away (indifferent to whatever nonsense you were preaching). I was trying to survive, and the lofty goal of being magnanimous was stratospherically out of reach. My needs for safety, security, love, were not being met and so I had no room in my life to live healthfully, but this was the point in my life where I needed a healthy mind, body, and spirit more than any other point in life. I needed help but was not able to actively pursue it. Like me, those who do not have their needs met try to survive day to day, but they need thoughtful and effective passive public health strategies for the long term. That way, they can reap the benefits without being

"Of the people, by the people, for the people" - Abraham Lincoln

asked to do anything out of the ordinary. As these policies start to add up—including viable medical insurance for all—we will begin to see more and more deprived American communities thriving, chasing their dreams, and giving more to the collective good than what they take because their dreams are the same as yours (love, safety, security, children), and now their basic human need for health care has been met, thus giving them the freedom to achieve. This will take bold leadership and responsibility, and then, perhaps, everyone in America will genuinely claim the right to life, liberty, and the pursuit of happiness. Perhaps, as we can make progress toward a just society, inclusive of all, we will collectively eschew the unjust society where the upwardly mobile unintentionally elevate themselves at the expense of the poor.

It has taken years to seal the hole I made in Iraq. It was not easy and still requires a daily renewed commitment. The medical hole, or the gap, that currently exists between the affluent and the less affluent must be closed—not only for their sake but for all our sakes. We often think that health care for all will drain our government's coffers even further and the social costs will be enormous. On the contrary, the costs of the current state of disenfranchisement of the poor are immeasurable. And as the system continues to collapse under the weight of its exclusionary policies, the ill effects will reverberate for decades. We need leadership, now, from those who are not afraid of doing the unpopular thing in order to have a sustainable and fiscally solvent future.

So, will we continue to make a hole that separates us? Or do we make an effort to change by filling it with policies that are

"Of the people, by the people, for the people" - Abraham Lincoln

good for all instead of just the privileged? Will we be "cool, calm, and collected" as we approach this topic in a measured tone or will we continue to stand on our ill-informed, emotional, and exclusionary soap-box, espousing nonsense that can't be backed up with actual facts?

My hope for writing this book is not to have a bunch of people agree with me on anything. My hope is that you will put the book down, start doing a little research for yourself, and then have an informed opinion on not only your own health but also the health of our country. That's it. My whole goal of this book is to get you to research what would happen if our great nation thoughtfully and deliberately offered universal health care to every one of our citizens. I think you will be surprised at the health care other countries can offer under a system of universal health care, and I think your opinion will shift and maybe, just maybe, you will shake your head at the never-ending rhetoric we hear out of our so-called news media and politicians when they talk about health care. They ought to be ashamed of themselves, because the game they are playing by delivering half-truths meant to give them secondary gain is killing people in active and passive ways.

To that end, it is only fair that I now tell you how for years I mistakenly felt like I utterly and completely failed as a doctor, officer and human when I decided to let an Iraqi die so that I could help an injured Marine instead. For years, I beat myself up over this situation because a **doctor** in war is not supposed to take sides—we took an oath to "first do no harm" and are supposed to treat the most injured first, regardless if they were a friend or foe. But I was also a **naval officer** whose job was to take care of

"Of the people, by the people, for the people" - Abraham Lincoln

the men and women of our military. The tension between these two roles, along with my being a conditional pacifist, produced a situation rife with conflict over obeying the oath of medicine or the duties of an officer. Finally, after years of perspective I realized that the horrible story of Chapter 6 is both my most shameful moment in life and the moment that gives me the courage to tackle health care now. For years I was wrongfully beating myself up over a situation that had no "right" or "moral" course of action. At the end of the day, I did the best I could. And that, my friends, is all any of us can ask.

The story of Chapter 6 was hard to write and will likely be hard to read. The story echoed a guilt that I should not have owned for over a decade. Now, this guilt is fueling me to lead this country, in whatever way I can, to a healthy future. Now the guilt is useful. For too long I held on to a false and too simplistic interpretation of an event in Iraq. Now, a little older and a little wiser, I see it for what it is. And I invite you to do the same. Have the courage to let your previous thoughts about health care be just that, your previous thoughts. Then give yourself the permission and freedom to research for yourself how universal health care works in other countries and perhaps admit that you were ill informed once, too. But do me a favor, frame Chapter 6 in the context of this chapter and ask yourself if our politicians, and us by proxy since we voted them into office, are intentionally and unintentionally turning their backs on the "have-nots" simply because they are the "haves."

Perhaps it is time to *"Make a hole!"* in our public health policy and realize that we are all in this together, that we are all dignified

"Of the people, by the people, for the people" - Abraham Lincoln

human beings who deserve good, affordable, and available health care so that we are left to chase after a destiny of our own choosing. We just have to choose leadership over partisanship, unrelenting bravery over dogmatic cowardice. It really is as simple as asking ourselves to whom we owe our loyalty and faithfulness: to political parties whose temper tantrums are well past pathetic or to a commitment to country that forges a strong and healthy future for our children, and our children's children, to thrive in the land of the free, home of the brave. For me, I choose commitment to country.

Semper Fidelis!

AFTER ACTION REVIEW:

- Put the book down and do a Google Search for "Universal Health Care" and start reading some articles. I do not want to ask you to go to a specific article because that would be leading the conversation. Instead, just read a few from reputable sources. I think you will be surprised at what you learn.

- Do a Google Search for "active and passive health policy" and dive into this subject a little deeper. The articles are fascinating and they might just inspire you to action, in maybe a passive way!

"Of the people, by the people, for the people" - Abraham Lincoln

NOTES:

NOTES:

CHAPTER 6

HOW TO MURDER NONVIOLENCE

"I was no party man myself, and the first wish of my heart was, if parties did exist, to reconcile them."
-George Washington

I WAS A CONDITIONAL pacifist before medical school. I attended an ecumenical seminary in Vancouver, Canada while studying Muay Thai Kickboxing and Wing Chun Kung Fu—not only to rid myself of the fear of physical pain, but also to understand and negate violence. We're all brothers and sisters in humanity, so why fight? There must be a better way to solve our problems; however, in order to preach nonviolence, I needed to see the other side of it.

Going to medical school meant taking on a lot more debt than I was willing to stomach, and since I grew up as a military brat, I knew ways to avoid that kind of weight. I decided it would be the wisest choice to join the military, have them pay for medical school, get an education and life experience, and then I would transition to civilian medicine. I didn't mind joining the military that has, at times, a violent mission, because doctors heal—they don't kill. It all made sense...in a very nonsensical way that only

20-something-year-olds can understand. After my internship (the first year after medical school), I had the choice of continuing in a residency program or doing an operational tour. I chose the latter, reasoning that there would never be another chance like this to experience the military for what it is, and I knew that wisdom would be invaluable.

MARINE RECON IT WAS

My father, a retired Lieutenant Colonel of the U.S. Air Force, told me that if Recon did not kill me, the experience would define the rest of my life and would make me stronger than perhaps anything else I could possibly do, in the military or perhaps even as a civilian. He was correct, in good and bad ways, as shattering your worldview is never an easy or clean process. But shattering your worldview is absolutely necessary to give one the wisdom and perspective that can only come with well-earned and thoroughly experienced blood, sweat, and tears.

We all know someone who espouses beliefs but cannot support them. Turn on TV and watch what passes as "news" today and you will have more examples than you can shake a stick at. We can't, nor should we, take them seriously as they have not earned the right to be heard and they never will, as long as what they continue to do is represent the half-truths that support their way of thinking while self-righteously pointing fingers of accusation at anyone who disagrees with their very convenient half-lies. These individuals are easily and understandably ignored because they are ineffectual, uninformed and disingenuous. Their book-smarts have no street-smarts to back them up, because for a theory to be proven, it must be practiced. So for me, I knew I had to earn the "street cred" around nonviolence and violence so that one day I could have a reasoned, balanced, and steady outlook.

My heroes were/are nonviolent, incredible, timeless leaders: Jesus, Eleanor Roosevelt, Mahatma Gandhi, Martin Luther King Jr., Susan B. Anthony, and Nelson Mandela to name a few. These incredible people changed the world with humility and self-sacrifice, and that was the world in which I wanted to exist. I didn't want to alter my (convenient) nonviolent perspective. Still, some things are inevitable. The momentum behind them can't be stopped, so it didn't take long before this pacifist's stance, which took decades to cultivate, was not only called into question, it was bludgeoned to death in Iraq. The first part of this book is the story of how this happened while trying the best I can to get you, the reader, to understand that if we do not do something about our "health care" system in this great country, the inevitable consequences of decades of poor public health policy, as well as the momentum of an enormously unhealthy populace, will cause the system to collapse in ruin and with it our freedoms as we have come to enjoy them.

Often, our imaginations are worse than reality. Not so much in war and not so much when the collapse of our "health care" system occurs. Eventually, the horror is mundane, while joy goes unnoticed. For Iraq, I thought I was prepared for the worst scenarios, and I even had a plan when I heard that there were casualties coming into Fallujah Surgical from my own battalion. For the USA, I hope to correct our deficiencies before the system

"Of the people, by the people, for the people" - Abraham Lincoln

collapses under the excessive burdens we have placed upon it for decades and that are only getting more and more burdensome every single day. If we are not successful, eventually there will be a straw that breaks the camel's back of medicine. And when this happens it will force reactionary policies to quickly correct the catastrophic consequences. The only solution for me is to lead by example, be vulnerable in the hopes of educating, write this book, inspire others to become part of the solution, shout from the mountaintops and scream from the city streets that NOW is the time to throw aside partisan temper tantrums and LEAD instead of squabble, listen instead of point fingers, intelligently compromise when needed instead of falling on an ideological sword of our own creating, see the big picture and move toward health instead of destroy for disingenuous gain. ENOUGH IS ENOUGH.

In this light, the rest of this chapter is dedicated to telling you the story of: what happened when I let differences in ideology dictate whether or not an Iraqi I was working on during a trauma resuscitation would live or die; when I had a moment of temporary insanity, gripped my pistol, and could only see red while facing off my commanding officer at Fallujah Surgical after one of my own corpsmen was dying because of a mission he ordered and that I strongly objected to; and, when I saw/smelled/felt what happens when an insurgent's rocket hit a bus full of women and children. This is not a comfortable chapter by any means and I would honestly suggest that if you are younger than 18, please do not read it, or ask your parents to read it first as it touches on horrific realities of the human condition. For those older than 18, please read this chapter with the mindset of a rational human

"Of the people, by the people, for the people" - Abraham Lincoln

who likely has not walked a mile in my shoes. It's okay to be horrified, because these stories are horrific. You may automatically judge me and my actions. But most importantly, I urge you to think about not only how horrible these stories are, but WHY they are so horrible and WHY they happened. Then, think about what will happen in this country if we do not START DEMANDING THAT OUR POLITICIANS, *AND WE OURSELVES,* STOP THINKING ABOUT WHAT IS BEST FOR THEIR/OUR POLITICAL PARTY AND START DOING THEIR/OUR JOB AS *RATIONAL HUMANS AND AMERICANS* AND ASK WHAT IS BEST FOR THE COUNTRY, FOR OUR FELLOW BROTHERS AND SISTERS, AND FOR OURSELVES.

THE HORRORS OF THINGS POORLY SET IN MOTION

I arrived at Fallujah Surgical before the casualties did, preparing to take care of someone under my direct command, someone who was one of my corpsmen (basically a mix between a medical assistant and a physician assistant) whose job it was to save lives. A Marine helped HM2 (my corpsman's rank) out of the Humvee with his hand over his chest, using all his power to walk by himself into the trauma bay. Even though he had been shot in the chest he still insisted on walking on his own, mostly unassisted.

No exit wound, I thought, which meant that the bullet was still inside and that it had likely ricocheted off his internal organs, making lung and heart soup of his chest cavity. A through-and-through wound is clean compared to a bullet bouncing around inside. Who knows what it destroyed?

"Of the people, by the people, for the people" - Abraham Lincoln

HM2 was still awake and having a hard time breathing, and even though he was not yet to the point where he was actively dying, he soon would be. There were six of us ready to receive him, so we called for the portable x-ray machine to determine how much blood was in the chest cavity and to locate the bullet. We thought we had a few minutes for a test that would hopefully aid us in the resuscitation. We were wrong.

Though the x-ray came up normal, HM2 was already fading. We transfused blood, administered oxygen, and continued our initial assessment. His condition continued to depreciate. I ordered two chest tubes because, regardless of the x-ray, he was dying. To save him, we followed the Rules of Trauma:

1)   Nobody is dead until they are warm (normal body temperature) and dead. This rule is ancient, and something all doctors accept. Often in trauma the body will start to cool down because the metabolism is adversely affected by the injuries. When a body is not functioning at optimal body temperature, it loses warmth, which can throw absolutely everything else off (this has also led to patients being prematurely pronounced dead when they should have just been declared "cold").

2)   Nobody is dead until they have two chest tubes and are dead. When a traumatic resuscitation isn't going well, and there's no obvious explanation for why the patient is dying, you have to make sure they have a normal temperature and that they have a chest tube stabbed into each lung cavity to allow them to release pressure and to breathe. If air or fluid (blood in this case) starts to fill up the chest cavity, it will cre-

ate too much pressure, inhibiting the lungs from inflating or deflating...and if you can't move air, you're dead. Chest tubes are usually placed below and to the side of each nipple. The tube is inserted into your chest, so the air or fluid (usually blood) can escape—kind of like sticking a straw into a water balloon. There are two chest cavities, so we put one tube on the left side of the chest and one on the right side of the chest. Usually, this procedure is done when the patient is unconscious or at least heavily sedated, because cutting through the skin, then ripping through the muscle between the ribs, and then stabbing the chest with sharp tubes is excruciatingly painful. Imagine, for a moment, what it would feel like if someone stabbed you in the chest, sawed through the muscle between your ribs, and then squeezed a finger into the space to spread the tissue apart. Then imagine the pain of stretching your rib bones apart enough to insert a tube, and finally, a thrust through your chest wall with an implement that's about half the size of a garden hose. *Holy hell*—the pain must be about the worst thing a human can experience. In war, some things need to be done, no matter how much pain they inflict. HM2 needed two chest tubes emergently and we did not have the luxury of time to get him numb first, as he was literally about to die. Holy hell indeed.

RULE NUMBER ONE

"Nobody is dead until they are warm and dead."
For my first deployment, Rule Number One was conveniently ignored on one occasion, and it is still an instructive memory

on what the human condition is able to justify given the right amount of pressure, exerted for the right amount of time, under the right conditions. This story continues to hurt, because it is a story about a deliberately xenophobic act by a man at the end of his rope who decided to let another man die simply because he was different, had a different point of view, and was on the other side of the conflict. Harry Stack Sullivan said it best when he said, "We are all much more simply human than otherwise." And this story points out what happens when ideologies/points of view/differences get in the way of doing what is right.

It was a day like any other in Fallujah: we were welcomed to the day with rockets and mortar fire; we were tired, we were dirty; we missed home; and we would give just about anything for a moment of true peace. As usual, I was called to help with another one of the unending mass casualties that came pouring into Fallujah Surgical on an almost daily basis. During this mass casualty event, I took the worst of the injured men and tried to stabilize him for surgery. He had lost a lot of blood after getting shot, his body temperature was dropping (he was "cold"), and he was about to go into shock. But he was conscious. He was in agony knowing that, even with great timing and available resources, he might not make it off the table. We ordered blood, warmed him up, gave him warm IV fluids; kept the bleeding under control, and kept his airway stable. Trauma is a continual battle of assessing and re-assessing until all the problems are fixed. Only then will the patient start to recover.

Trauma resuscitations are chaotic. The incident absorbs your attention as there is a very sick person present, and their bodily fluids are everywhere. It makes surfaces slippery (right next to a collection of silvery, sharp objects). What's worse, there are unknown items on or in the person being treated, and with so much to do, there are too many cooks in the desert kitchen. A good trauma response relies on one essential, a leader who can manage the madness by assigning and tracking progress of specific tasks. One of my talents in life has always been to lead, no matter how confusing the situation, so when things started to devolve, I became better, more deliberate. I didn't crack with the pressure; instead, I thrived with hidden variables. To watch me work during a code was motivating for those around me because my mindset was always, *Give me more—we have not even begun the real challenge.* That's my arena. Needless to say, I was always very good at resuscitating trauma victims, at least when my heart was in it. And in trauma resuscitations, if your heart and soul are not in it to win it, people die. This time, for this patient, I just did not care if he lived or died. And if the leader (or our political leaders when it comes to health care) does not care, people die. The trauma victim and I were in essence on opposite "sides of the aisle"; it was easy for me to be self-righteous and not be a rational, thoughtful, and caring human whose job it was to save lives, to heal, to make people's lives better with my talents and skills. Honestly, I just did not care about this trauma resuscitation; I just wanted this asshole to die so I could move on.

The next most injured person was ten feet away, and while not anywhere close to stable, he was not nearly as bad as my patient. But that's where I wanted to be; that was the patient I wanted to treat; he was the one I wanted to live. The problem

"Of the people, by the people, for the people" - Abraham Lincoln

was that my patient was an Iraqi insurgent who had just shot the Marine ten feet away. The Marine was "on my side," one of my own, thought like me, behaved like me, had a similar upbringing, believed many of the same things I did... The Iraqi was the "enemy" who was not "on my side," was not "one of my own," did not think like me, did not behave like me, did not have a similar upbringing to mine, did not believe many of the same things I did... We were different and therefore he was able to be objectified, vilified, and ultimately left there to die on the table.

How is it that a Marine is over there and I'm here, helping the fucker who shot one of us when all we are trying to do in this God-forsaken country is help them?

And in what fucked-up world is the enemy the priority?!?

And if you are reading this and thinking how horrible this section is: 1) *You have no idea what it was like to be in war and what it does to you;* and 2) YOU ARE COMPLETELY CORRECT. IT IS HORRIBLE. And it's my most shameful moment. The Iraqi's life was not expendable. **There is no "*Us vs. Them.*"** Regardless, this is the truth about my failure. It would have been a violation of the Hippocratic and Osteopathic oaths to which I swore—the actions of a man at the end of his rope.

In a mass casualty event, time compresses and decisions that are made have immediate impact. And in war, you know who is jeopardizing your own life and the life of those you care about and you can address that, usually very quickly. In the civilian health care world, decisions can take a long time to develop and their impact may also take a long time to manifest in enough numbers that their impact, intended or not, can be measured.

"Of the people, by the people, for the people" - Abraham Lincoln

And in civilian life, those people making health care policy are some group(s) that you can't talk to, don't see, and besides all that, are sometimes immune from the same policies they are forcing on you, as is the case for members of Congress who have their own "Cadillac" health care plans that "common" citizens can't even access. Because of all these factors, most Americans are sort of like the frog in a slowly heating up pot of water. Things happen that they don't understand and it happens incrementally, so there's no perceived immediate need for action as is the case in war or in a mass casualty event. But in both cases, health care and life itself are immediately or eventually impacted in big ways and small.

In a mass casualty event, especially in wartime, the decision on whom to treat first can be complicated by who the patient is—one of "us" or one of "them" (the enemy). Ideally, a doctor shouldn't think about "us" or "them." A patient needs help and that patient gets it. End of story. But like many things in life, what is ideal isn't always what happens, and this is exacerbated if emotions (fear, anger, hate, frustration), exhaustion, politics, bureaucracy, or money are involved.

I fell into just this situation in Iraq, and while this incident may not seem related to health care in America, it is, because it illustrates in the time-compressed reality of combat medicine what can happen in America—indeed what IS happening in America—if decisions on who should have access to or receive health care are polluted by the factors mentioned above.

My mind was swimming. The patient smelled, he wore Iraqi clothes, and he didn't speak my language. He was a dirty fucking piece of shit who attacked us. We were not the same. We couldn't be more dissimilar while ten feet away, a Marine, wearing the same uniform as I, thinking the same way I thought, coming from a similar culture and background as I did, was in pain and being resuscitated by other medical assets at Fallujah Surgical.

Fuck this Iraqi motherfucker.

Let him die.

I halfheartedly gave the Iraqi patient blood and stabilized him as quickly and as poorly as possible, because time was vital and I wanted to help resuscitate my "brother-in-arms" instead. The asshole on my table was an enemy who came for us. Fuck him.

Wasn't he the source of all of this suffering?!

While we liberated the Iraqi people from an oppressive regime, they were killing us as their thanks. None of us wanted to be here. None of us wanted to fight in a war in which we didn't believe. Hot, sweaty, and homesick, we put ourselves in harm's way—on purpose—and for what?

Goddamn this whole shit-sandwich of a fucked-up mess.

Fuck this assclown who injured the people trying to help him.

Fuck him.

Okay, so he is hurt and shot and about to die.

That's what you get.

That is what you deserve, and the quicker it happens, the faster I can help the "good guys."

Rot in hell, shithead.

While in the middle of the Iraqi's resuscitation, I never even came close to committing my mind, talents, and resources to saving his life. Quite the reverse. Distracted by everything going

"Of the people, by the people, for the people" - Abraham Lincoln

on with the other trauma team, I listened for commotion, for cries of anguish carried down the hall as other Marines were being triaged and resuscitated. The Iraqi moaned on the table, but I was more annoyed than concerned by his vocalizations of pain and suffering. What was concerning was that his whining kept me from focusing on concrete details just ten feet away.

Trauma is an all or nothing game, and if you are not present, then you are worse than worthless—you are dangerous to the patient and the team.

Damn it!

To top it all off, we were taking incoming mortars and rockets. While there were no direct hits on our building, the walls shook, paint fell from the ceiling, and all sorts of dust and debris were dislodged from this makeshift facility, floating through the air. Not good.

Fuck this God-forsaken shithole.

Camp Fallujah was under attack for the third time this day. Yes, we were normally shot at multiple times a day, but I wasn't yet 100 percent used to people trying to kill me or the percussion from bomb blasts, and the explosions really didn't motivate me to treat the dying Iraqi in front of me. I mean, "his people" were trying to kill us while I was sort of trying to save one of their own. Adrenaline flowed through me as dust sifted off the ceiling. Then, the whole building shook (and, in case you were wondering, dust-coated trauma victims are not exactly a sterile or appropriate environment in which to conduct a trauma resuscitation). The environment wasn't suitable for stitches. How was I going to save somebody in it—

"Of the people, by the people, for the people" - Abraham Lincoln

Fuck this place.

God-fucking-shit-damn-it.

Fuck it! Fuck this patient. Fuck this war.

I'm out. This piece of shit can die.

I stopped working on the Iraqi and told the others to stop their efforts, before walking away.

The policy was that when a doctor decides to stop a trauma resuscitation or pronounce a patient dead, it needs to be confirmed by another doctor, in case something was forgotten. In this case, I had forgotten to show up and do my best. Fortunately, even in war there are checks and balances, so when I approached the other doctor and presented the case, it went something like this:

"Multiple gunshot trauma in shock. Two liters of blood transfused, labored breathing, hypotensive, pulse declining, unconscious, and hypothermic at seventy-five degrees. Calling the code." I recited the information quickly—in a tone that was not asking permission. I was telling the other doctor what was happening and that we were just going to allow the asshole to die.

"Not intubated?" my colleague asked. Intubation is when a tube is put down the throat and into the lungs so that we can breathe for the patient when they are unable to do so on their own. It's standard in trauma, and in the world where I still gave a shit, it would have already been done.

"No. He's maintaining his airway and breathing adequately, although that's declining. He's decompensating, and we do not have the resources to continue when there are others who need our help."

What a load of shit!

He was barely breathing and "barely" was nowhere near what his body needed.

"Cold?"

"Yup. Seventy-five-degree core temperature."

"Not dead until warm and dead."

"Wasting resources. Others need help."

"Not dead until warm and dead," the doc repeated.

"How long am I going to waste my time on this? He is already dead!"

"Not dead until warm and dead."

Yeah, he was right; however, at that moment, I wanted to slap him and tell him to grow the fuck up.

After a five-second stare-down, I figured I ought to at least go back and work on the patient a little longer—until the inevitable happened.

I turned and continued with the resuscitation. After having been called out, I started to work the code as I should have, and within three minutes, he was warm, somewhat conscious, and stable enough for surgery. Three minutes of my actually giving a shit was all it took. The other doctor glanced over at me and nodded, knowing that he just saved two humans: the Iraqi and me, because I would have never let it go if I let him die. My only regret now is that if I had skipped the whole insolent ass-holic behavior on my part, that would have translated into more time for the Marines who needed me. I did not give one shit that this man's life was saved. All I cared about was that I could finally move on.

Live or die, asshole—I don't care.

"Of the people, by the people, for the people" - Abraham Lincoln

A physician's mission in war is to treat anyone who needs help. There is no favoritism or preferential treatment for your comrades, which is a solid tenet of care that I support; without this rule, triage would be squarely reduced to what side you fought for—and we would only treat the Iraqis after every single Marine was treated (even the ones who only needed a Band-Aid and maybe a juice box). This type of prejudice is criminal, and yet that is precisely, and most ashamedly, what I did. I do not think it was inherent bias. It was not about right or wrong. It was not politically motivated. It came down to primal mentality—the "Us vs. Them"—which is the same mindset that has encouraged every atrocity in the history of mankind, and the same mindset that makes it easy for our politicians to behave as they do towards each other and by proxy towards the country they are supposed to be leading. It is the reason for war. Whenever you turn an individual person into the "other," then you can do whatever you want and be justified.

Perhaps their nose is shaped differently. Perhaps their clothes are foreign. Or it's the way they speak, but there's always some criticism or rationalization that you can make to excuse your actions in the moment. Doctors, and politicians and citizens, must remain impartial, so when I made it personal, I was able to use the "logical" justification; there were simply "not enough resources" to support the animal inside of me. I almost bought my own lie, until the other doctor corrected me—I was not doing my job as a doctor or as a human. I was acting like a raging, selfish asshole with another person's life on the line, and this other doctor was my conscience. He was having none of it.

"Of the people, by the people, for the people" - *Abraham Lincoln*

Before people used "woke" as a buzzword, I'd always prided myself on not being a racist or a bigot or a sexist or—

Well, Reagan, it turns out that you too, in the midst of the fog of war, of exhaustion, and of being shot at, you also have your limit.

I let it get so bad that I regarded another human as disposable. Perhaps Rule Number One of Trauma should be changed. Maybe it should be: "Treat others how you would like to be treated...and don't be an asshole," or something like that.

And that was a defining moment for me and one of the driving factors for this book. As I returned back to my "normal" self, and then upon reflection on that day, it crystalized in me that not only could I do better, but that I also needed to recalibrate and bring into balance my idealism, my obligation to my Marines as a combat doctor, and my obligation as a physician towards all people, no matter their allegiance or anything other than the fact they are a human being who needs my help. It turns out, life isn't as black and white as I or many people would like it to be, and it is our fate as humans to have to navigate through the oftentimes gray and confusing landscape of life. And this is made more complicated considering the constant stream of propaganda and self-serving half-lies we are fed by the media, politicians, educators, etc. But the good news is we are all endowed with intellect and free will with which to reason things out for ourselves and then take action to redress bad policy or whatever. In wartime, the weapons to bring about change are typically bullets and bombs. In a rational civilian world, at least in the USA, our weapons for change are votes and pressure on elected officials to be rational (the reverse of "political") and think of

"Of the people, by the people, for the people" - Abraham Lincoln

public policy in terms of measurably benefitting the "PUBLIC," not just some segments of the public. I submit that there isn't any more far-reaching public policy that desperately needs rational thought and action than America's fractured health care system.

RULE NUMBER TWO

HM2

On the day my corpsman was shot, I cradled the 9mm pistol at my hip. Gripped by rage, all my polite and pretentious assertions were finally in their death-throes. The commanding officer was walking down the hall, concerned about the status of one of *his men*—a corpsman who was ordered into a compromising situation against my protests. This was the same commanding officer who wanted to provoke an attack and "shoot some bad guys."

When the commanding officer and I faced off in the hallway outside of the trauma bay where I had been working on one of *my men*, my hand slid to my holstered sidearm.

"How is HM2?" he asked. The anger flared, and my gaze transformed. From harsh to raw with hatred. I just stared back at him.

I'd never felt the power of rage before. My comfortable theories about life, God, civility, nonviolence, and purpose were quickly ravaged by pride, hate, adrenaline, and contempt. Blood—like hot, smelting iron—ravaged my veins. There was nothing else in the hallway filled with the commotion of a mass casualty. For he and I were about to engage. There was nothing else in my soul. There was nothing left of me as a rational human, a doctor, an officer, a son…nothing but pure unaltered hatred and rage.

"Of the people, by the people, for the people" - Abraham Lincoln

ONE DAY PRIOR

A day earlier, I was in a command and staff meeting preparing for the mission that resulted in HM2 being shot, and the battalion had to come together. Recon BN is supposed to be the baddest of the bad, the tip of the spear, the Marines you send for when you need a whole lot of shit destroyed without asking twice. However, we were not getting much "business" in Fallujah, because we had a reputation and few dared to engage us face to face. An Iraqi insurgent, or most any other fighting force on the planet, would have very little chance of survival if he took on Recon Marines straight up. Therefore, the Iraqis resorted to IEDs they could hide in the dirt so we would drive over them, and rockets and mortars they could shoot at us from a distance. In response to this lack of face-to-face engagement, we started doing more and more things to provoke attacks. Our "kill sheet" hadn't had any numbers added to it recently; Recon was getting restless.

Every command and staff meeting included a contest between the different companies in the battalion. Recon BN was divided into three equal companies of Recon Marines, and inside each company, they were divided further. All three companies were in competition, of course, but instead of comparing how many push-ups or sit-ups they could do, it was all about "confirmed kills." Now, these confirmed kills did not necessarily have to be of enemy combatants (as one would logically think)—they just had to be "Iraqi souls that were set free." And as far as I know, the different battalions within the region reported these numbers to the generals who kept track of who were the best "killers." Of course, Recon had to, by definition, be the best at killing since we were the baddest of the bad and we had a reputation to protect.

Recon BN was well-known in Fallujah, and when we rolled into an area, the enemy took the day off because they knew that we would "Cry 'Havoc!' and let slip the dogs of war." After seeing this battalion in action, I think Shakespeare had us in mind when he thought of "dogs of war." Recon BN was brutally and skillfully efficient in mass destruction on a biblical scale. But when there was no one to fight, Recon had to do something to get our numbers up. So, we did stupid shit to put us at a considerable tactical disadvantage, so hopefully, the "bad guys" would think the odds were in their favor, and they'd come out to play.

For example, I remember a particular mission heading back to Camp Fallujah in the middle of the night after a "boring" mission (no confirmed kills). Given the lack of action, our company commander decided to drive into the center of a very hostile town, stop the Humvees in the middle of the street with buildings surrounding us, while blaring Godsmack music at a perversely loud volume at two in the morning. We stood in the street waiting to get shot at. We were easy targets in a very compromising position, and yet, for a good fifteen minutes, we couldn't see anyone in the surrounding buildings. I wondered how long it would take for the bullets and rockets to fly. We were terrorizing this town, and no one responded because they knew we were Recon; they knew that, even with the tactical advantage of the high ground and our being out in the open between buildings, engagement meant that we'd come down on them with vengeful fury. Eventually, we left, storming off like the bullies we were, and headed back to Camp Fallujah without any confirmed kills for the mission.

In another instance, Recon BN was so bored that they decided to stage another stupid mission (in which, look vulnerable enough to tempt the enemy into a firefight), which would add some more confirmed kills to the sheet. In their finite wisdom, however, they decided that I would venture into the outskirts of Fallujah—an area that was particularly violent—and medically treat the locals. I was excited at first. I wanted to help people, but as they detailed the mission, it was apparent that they were going to be using the sick and injured to lure the Iraqis out to fight. They planned to drive into town, announcing that the Americans would be there to help the ill and injured at a specific location and time the next day. The sick would come, and so would the fighters. I should observe that it's never a brilliant strategy to tell your adversary the time and place for a convenient attack, but that's Recon for you. The plan does not have to make sense! It just needs to result in confirmed kills. I was furious that they were planning to use my patients to bait the Iraqi fighters into our own ambush.

In what world is it advantageous to use the ill, injured, and infirm to provoke a firefight?!

Well...one in which the other side doesn't matter.

Since I was technically Navy (and not a Marine), I went outside the leadership of Recon BN, to my Navy medical commanding officer, and asked for his help to stop an unnecessarily dangerous, reckless and amoral mission, in my opinion. While there was nothing he could do, I had a choice: bow out or submit. If

I disobeyed a direct command, then I'd be court-martialed and leave Recon BN without a doctor again, and the mission would still go ahead as planned. Or, if I complied, then I could try to bring some sanity to a senseless situation. I complied.

A foot patrol went out the night before to get the lay of the land. I went along. It was a beautiful night, and for a very brief moment, it felt like a peaceful hike. We wound up in the mayor's house, where locals streamed in to see me. They knew we were coming, so they were actively bringing in their sick; the problem was that the local fighters also knew we were coming. When I saw who they brought for treatment, it broke my heart because all I really had was my trauma bag—nothing for chronic conditions. In the middle of the night, there was no way to know if the waiting people meant us harm or not. Not having any supplies, apart from those used to patch up gunshot wounds, I did the best I could. On the way to the compound we had commandeered, the Marines thought it would be funny to put me with our Iraqi interpreter whom we met earlier that day. As we walked back, we were separated from each other by 150 yards—close enough to mostly see the Marines near us, but too far away to hear each other unless we yelled really loudly. It was sketchy since I had no idea if the interpreter had my back or not. Essentially, he and I were walking back to the compound, in enemy territory, just barely within eyesight of the Marines. It was a torment to wonder, *how much would I be worth if he managed to separate me from the group and abduct me?*

We walked back to our makeshift compound for forty-five minutes; there were many points when I did not see another

Marine for an extended period. After we arrived in relative safety, I met with the corpsmen to discuss the next day's planned insanity.

During this mission, the medical assets would be set in the center of the road, allowing the locals to approach from up and down the road. On the neighboring rooftop, Recon snipers with .50 caliber sniper rifles waited for insurgents to attack. Medevac helicopters were standing by to receive the wounded. A few of my corpsmen and I stood out in the open, practicing makeshift medicine. It was sheer ridiculousness, and I am happy to report that no one died that day. I was not able to deliver any real medicine, but at least it was not a bloodbath. These are just a few examples of what Recon BN did when they were bored and when their kill sheet columns were empty.

RULE NUMBER TWO

HM2

The HBO Special, based on the exploits of Recon BN during the initial push into Iraq, was titled *Generation Kill*. There's a reason for that. Recon is a hammer, which only has one purpose, and when a hammer is your best tool, everything looks like a nail. When planning the mission in which HM2 was shot, in the face of reason they chose to risk my men—men under my direct command as the Officer in Charge of the medical department— just to tempt insurgents into the open. What I feared would happen, did happen, and one of my corpsmen, HM2, was shot; others were also injured.

Since I didn't go on this mission, I was at Camp Fallujah when

"Of the people, by the people, for the people" - Abraham Lincoln

Fallujah Surgical called and said that there was another mass casualty coming in—except this time, it was with men from my battalion. My heart sank. *Please let this be just a nightmare.* I had purposely distanced myself from everyone in Recon BN because I needed to remain objective if I was going to have any success when it came to saving them; however, I also had to be close enough to the men to see when the fog of war was too thick, they were too complacent, and their heads simply weren't in the game. I accomplished this with miniature, daily conversations; based on their reactions, I could evaluate their psychological wellbeing. I could help them concentrate on staying frosty, because most of the Marines who were injured in Iraq were not injured because the enemy was overly smart, or prepared, or equipped. We hurt ourselves—either by doing something stupid or losing focus—and we paid for our inattention in carnage. But HM2 was under my command and I spent a lot of time with the medical assets of Recon BN because I had to train them, mentor them, manage them. I knew HM2 too well and I was horrified that he was one of the casualties, absolutely terrified that I would not be able to objectively treat someone whom I knew so well; he might die under my care as I could no longer be objective during his resuscitation. This had to be a nightmare and I would wake up anytime soon. *Please God, don't let this be real.*

I arrived at Fallujah Surgical a few minutes before the casualties, which gave me the chance to figure out who all of the casualties were and who the most injured likely were. I knew them all well. Somehow, I had to find a way to compartmentalize my

"Of the people, by the people, for the people" - Abraham Lincoln

emotions so they wouldn't affect my treatment. This has always been a struggle for me—so much so that, during cadaver labs in medical school, I had to excuse myself from every single one because I couldn't be in front of people. I needed to be alone to contemplate, and pay reverence to, the life of the person I was dissecting. Separating the corpse from the real person was difficult. Separating my corpsmen from their wounds would be an impossibility.

When the Humvee rolled up, HM2 got out of the vehicle and tried to walk on his own into Fallujah Surgical. This combat-hardened corpsman was shot in the chest and still had the pride of wanting to walk in on his own. He insisted on it and even though he was mortally wounded, no one dared take his pride away by putting him on a stretcher. He walked proud and strong. A Marine was supporting him, and after he had traveled most of the way and it was apparent that he was completely unable to take another wobbly step, we put him on a stretcher and brought him back into the trauma bay. Other than the single entry wound, he did not seem to sustain any other injuries. Young and in shape, his body was able to compensate for a short while. I feared that meant he would destabilize quickly, and though we ordered the tests and started to stabilize him, our efforts proved to be useless. He started to crash.

There was one thing left to do—insert chest tubes and decompress his chest—only, there was no time to anesthetize the area. As such, we had to complete the procedure without numbing medication. This was going to hurt, a lot.

Though HM2 was starting to decompensate, he was still alert

and oriented, and he locked eyes on me when he heard what was about to happen. I wasn't the one who needed to do the procedure. I was the one who needed to hold his hand while staring him down so that he knew that he was not alone. For several minutes, our fists interlocked. He was stabbed, his ribs were torn open, and then we punched a tube into his lungs. Stoic and locked in place, we had made a tunnel into each other's soul, and I do not think either of us would ever be able to forget these tormented minutes of the procedure. HM2 had many great and admirable qualities but I never knew just how tough he was. Few people on the planet could have taken that procedure like he did. He was a hardened warrior with the heart of an American—and neither one of those dies easily.

Over a liter of blood poured out of his left lung. We knew that he had to go to surgery instantly. This was shocking because the chest x-ray was so shitty that we could not see a liter of blood in his lungs! That is how bad our medical equipment was. Within three minutes, he was in the surgical suite and emergently prepped for surgery. I left him there and went out to care for the others. When I went back into the surgical suite, though, I was horrified. The surgeons were having a hard time controlling the bleeding, and they couldn't see what they were working on. Every part of me wanted to push them aside and take over because they were reacting, not thinking. It was like a scene from a bad horror film. One of the surgeons shoved his hand inside HM2's chest, grabbed a chunk of lung and blood clot, yanked it out, and then threw it into a bucket.

What the fuck are you thinking?!

"Of the people, by the people, for the people" - Abraham Lincoln

You don't blindly put your hand into a chest and yank out whatever you find.

This isn't noodling!

I didn't know what to do. On one hand, it was evident that they were in over their heads and did not have the training, poise, support, facilities, or equipment they needed; really, they were doing the best they could under horrible conditions. On the other hand, they were panicking. I didn't have the training to take over, but at least I had my wits.

Fuck.

I walked out of the surgical suite, hoping against reason that the doctors would regain their composure and save HM2's life. I was shaking with fear, anger, hopelessness, guilt, and rage. Pure rage. That's the moment I looked up to see my commanding officer coming toward me, and all I saw was red. Red, hot flowing blood coming from his head. The concept of "temporary insanity" had seemed like a convenient excuse to commit a crime, and not a real condition—that is, until I experienced it.

Wrath and hatred were rioting inside me, and that overwhelmed everything else I felt. Strength seemed to surge in my muscles, making me invincible. Yes, the commanding officer was also a man I respected. He was my patient, a fellow American, and I thought he was the right choice for the job (in fact, both of my commanding officers at Recon BN were very good leaders, good Marines, and good men in my opinion). It was an honor to serve with him, but in this rage-induced frenzy, I wanted to hurt whoever was responsible for HM2's present condition. However, the person who was accountable was dead on the battlefield. The only one left to blame was the commanding officer walking toward me, looking concerned.

With my hand on top of my 9mm pistol attached to my right thigh, with HM2's blood on my combat fatigues, with a guilty and exhausted convoluted mess of a conscience, I looked at the commanding officer without a thought in my head. There was nothing. Flat-lined. I was not a rational human. I was reduced to animal instincts of pure ego, boiling over, overwhelmed, and lusting to retaliate at somebody, not that he deserved any of it. He felt as bad as, if not worse than I did. I could see it in his eyes and in his stature. Besides, I was also his doctor. He needed to have the freedom to come to me whenever he needed help, but instead of an ally, the commanding officer met an adversary in that hallway—one who had already judged him. I was too far gone to be empathetic, though. All I wanted was an eye for an eye.

Fortunately, for both of us, my chief (administrative head of my medical department) saw that shit was about to go south, so he came out of the adjoining room, and put his arm around me without asking the commanding officer to excuse us. Chief, with his arm around my neck, forcibly pulled me away without saying a word. He just needed time and space to keep my rage contained, as he was experienced and wise enough to know when someone no longer had a rational thought left in his head. Chief sat with me, not saying a word, just staring directly into my eyes, hoping that I would wake up from this rage-induced stupor if I saw a familiar face. After a few minutes, my rational mind would return; only then would I be able to brief my commanding officer of HM2's status. By the grace of God, the surgeons were able to stabilize him. I was eventually able to briefly inform the commanding officer of HM2's status.

HM2 was medevaced to Baghdad for additional surgeries and care, and while his left lung was almost destroyed, HM2 lived!!!

Thank you, God. Thank you, thank you, thank you—

After the mass casualty and everything was cleaned up at Fallujah Surgical, I went to the gym and started lifting. Disoriented, I did bicep curls well past failure, not realizing that my nerves were screaming for me to stop. The adrenaline overflowed, making me numb, so I pushed it until a pop vibrated through me, and then the heavyweight crashed down. Something in my right elbow had snapped, and I still wake up from the residual pain (even though the wound should have healed over a decade ago). It has been fourteen years since the incident, yet no matter what I do, the pain that engulfed this moment is not something that I can—or probably should—get over. Some injuries are unrecoverable, and they're meant to warn us about events that could be prevented. That way, we don't allow them to happen again. And the more of us who carry with us these soul wounds, the less likely that we will engage in vain. It's a scar worth keeping.

War is ugly. It pushed me to the edge of an irrevocable sin—to assault my commanding officer. My nonviolent philosophies could not withstand a trauma resuscitation on one of my men who was foolishly placed in harm's way. I was still reeling when they called me to Fallujah Surgical a couple of weeks later, and while there had been other calls, they were typical traumas (whatever that means). By this time, my heart had become so calloused to war that I reacted to mass casualties with all the emotion of brushing my teeth. As I walked to Fallujah Surgical, I noticed that I was no longer in a hurry. I was finally "cool, calm and collected," but it was not because I finally understood what this meant and decided to conduct myself accordingly. It was because I was flat-lined in every emotional sense possible.

When I arrived, the scent of burning flesh hit me like a wall. Burned skin, muscles, sinew, and scorched hopes and dreams. The insurgents hit a school bus full of women and children with a rocket. And, inside, there were remains of some U.S. military as well as Iraqi women and children. The bodies were no longer inside the bus, though. They were a part of it, melted into the seats and the floor. Everyone was dead.

I do not remember anything else about that day or many of the days that came thereafter. There is a black hole of memories that will likely come alive and haunt me in the future, as is apt to happen to veterans when dementia sets in, but there's something that's quite clear: I distinctly remember wanting to rip the insurgents apart, limb by painful limb with my bare hands. I wanted them to pay. I'd make it painful and prolonged for this, as well as every other horrible thing they had done. Finally, I realized that there are instances in which the best answer is also the most violent one—to call in the hammer and salt the earth with their blood because they have no hope of ever being "human." Sometimes, a violent hammer like Recon BN can bring the medicine the world needs to heal by murdering evil; as far as I was concerned, there was no more consternation about the nature, or the usefulness, of hammers, of violence. Violence now was acceptable in certain circumstances, for certain people who had revoked their right to be treated as human ever again.

Although very infrequently, I do acknowledge that there is an element of society that has lost its right to be a part of the world. Whosoever is capable of murdering a bus full of innocent women and children must submit his right to freedom and, in my opinion, needs to be put down like a rabid dog. Pure pacifism was no longer an option for me. Pure violence is also not an option for me. There are seasons for both. Similarly, I find myself not being on the "left" or the "right" of any situation anymore. Instead, I see nuances to most problems that are not dealbreakers; in fact, those nuances are the inherent difficulties that are needed to craft sound policies, epistemologies, and rubrics. When there is an easy answer, it is almost always wrong, and just as nonviolence has its limitations, so does violence. Like most things in life, an extreme position on either side of the pendulum, or aisle, negates common sense. There is a place for each and a whole world of nuanced situations in the middle that must be governed by common sense instead of radicalism.

THE CORRELATION TO PUBLIC HEALTH

The divide between Republicans and Democrats is more exaggerated than ever. If there is anything that the current political climate is teaching us, it is that when we isolate ourselves from someone, labeling them "other," we put our need for "security" and the "rule of law" above human rights and basic common sense. Then, we can justify horrific actions, ineffectual policies, and a dogmatism which will place the argument above the greater good. The mindset of "Us vs. Them" allowed me to put a null value on an Iraqi's life. I would've let him die, and I am immensely ashamed of that lapse in my sound judgment but I do understand why it happened in the middle of the chaos. Now, the same thing is happening in our country; it's equally shameful when individuals, whether they be politicians or ordinary citizens, swear themselves to their political parties or ideologies and forget that we are a government for the people, by the people, and of the people. We must not label ourselves Republicans, Democrats, or... We are Americans who should be loyal to American ideals; instead, we subscribe to the party dogma, excusing the inexcusable and perpetuating a broken system of people pointing fingers at each other instead of being actively engaged in leading this great country.

There was a study about how labels drive us apart and discourage us from thinking critically. The study was of a fake legislative bill that was shown to Democrats and Republicans. Everything was identical about the bill except for at the top, where they wrote that it was authored by either a Democrat or a Republican. When Republicans read the bill that was supposedly written by a Republican, they all liked it and all the Democrats did not like it. But when it was said to be written by a Democrat, all of the Republicans now did not like it and all the Democrats did. But, the only thing that changed in this fake bill was who they thought wrote it/supported it. Only the label mattered. The content was inconsequential. This is a big problem.

"A house divided cannot stand." (Mark 3:25) These ancient words of wisdom are just as valid today as when they were written

"Of the people, by the people, for the people" - Abraham Lincoln

in antiquity. George Washington warned us in his farewell address that the divisiveness of political parties will eventually destroy the USA, as the natural tendency of man is to bend toward entropy, rather than cohesiveness. He warned that ultimately, it would become more important to belittle and destroy the opposing party than it will be to unite the country. Does this sound familiar?

This divide is supported and perpetuated by the media, whose ratings are spurred by contention, whose viewers start thinking that it's acceptable to behave poorly towards each other, to not listen to each other, to belittle instead of finding common ground, being divisive instead of united, being polarized instead of exercising good old-fashioned common sense. The media gets us enraged, worried and not encouraged to help or be helpful. The media knows that if they can just get us angry and not talking to anyone who has a different point of view, they will have all the power. We yell when we should listen. We leave someone to die instead of resuscitating him. Had another physician not reminded me of who I am and what my commitments are, that man would have died. Similarly, if we do not come together with our collective interests in mind, then we will not make progress on anything, let alone the health of our great nation. If we keep listening to the media and modeling their poor example, instead of thinking for ourselves and reaching across the aisle to those who might disagree with us, then we will continue to be puppets of the media instead of thoughtful citizens. If our politicians keep acting like toddlers having a continual temper tantrum, our country will further slip and eventually fail altogether.

"Of the people, by the people, for the people" - Abraham Lincoln

Health care is at a crossroads. Without a concerted effort, the entire system will collapse in the next ten to fifteen years. Personally, I am surprised it has not done so already. Now is the time to find common ground and to examine how other countries handle their health care to see what, if any, policies might be appropriate for the USA. With their example, we can exploit the best practices and dismiss the ones that will not work for us. We need to create a system with a focus on prevention and education. Let ideas stand on their own merits. Let challenges guide nuanced and constructive debate. Let our love for each other and our country be stronger than our need to separate and sort by rank, because we are AmeriCANs, not AmeriCANTs. Let common sense start to rule the hallowed halls of this great nation.

We are the United States of America. Perhaps it is time that we stand together, perhaps with different points of view, with an eye for what is healthful for our country instead of just yelling at each other, trying to vie for power. Perhaps we need to talk to each other. Perhaps we need to get rid of this "Us vs. Them" mindset that puts brother against brother and sister against sister, and actually start talking to each other, actually start demanding that our media report the news instead of trying to spread their own propaganda, actually force our politicians to act like adults who are interested in the wellbeing of this great country instead of toddlers who only care about garnering more power at the expense of the country. Perhaps now, today, is the day that we the people stand up for our country and demand better of ourselves, the media, and our political system. Perhaps today, we the people start leading instead of being sheep led to

"Of the people, by the people, for the people" - Abraham Lincoln

the slaughter. Perhaps today, we figure out how to murder the partisan nonsense and start standing together, united, in the common goal and good of "country first."

United we stand,

Divided we...

AFTER ACTION REVIEW:

- Today, listen to someone who thinks differently than you about something. But, please do not say a word until they are finished and you are sure that you understand their position. Do not listen with an ear toward forming your own counter-argument. Just listen. Once you think you thoroughly understand their point of view, ask if you can express that back to them. If they agree that you under-stand their point of view, the assignment is done. DO NOT ENGAGE THEM WITH YOUR POINT OF VIEW UN-LESS THEY ASK FOR IT. Your assignment is just to listen and understand what someone else, who does not think like you, thinks. That is it. It will be harder than you think but so worth it. I think you will find that what they want, at the foundation of their argument, is exactly what you want: safety, security, love, health care. They just have a different thought about how to get there. THIS IS GOOD NEWS BECAUSE YOU BOTH WANT THE SAME THINGS!!!
- Write the media and your politicians and hold them ac-countable for their actions while not yelling at them for thinking what they think. Ask them to be honest brokers of the truth. Ask them to represent both sides fairly and with-

"Of the people, by the people, for the people" - Abraham Lincoln

out an agenda. Ask them to behave like the leaders they are and listen instead of yell. They will only change if we demand it, if we ourselves model it, and if we encourage it in others.

"Of the people, by the people, for the people" - Abraham Lincoln

NOTES:

NOTES:

Chapter 7

Memorial Day

"The past is prophetic in that it asserts loudly that wars are
poor chisels for carving out peaceful tomorrows."
-Martin Luther King Jr.

WHEN THE FOG of war set in, everything felt confusing. I was not alert, awake, or oriented. It was midafternoon and it was hot, 110+ degrees hot. All I knew was that we were on top of a building, supporting a sniper who had an enemy combatant in his sights. He was awaiting orders from our commanding officer to pass mortal judgment on another human.

I could see the enemy combatant, waiting just outside of a school on the top of another building; the children were about to be let out for the day, and he had leveled his rifle on the front door. There was something else—a detonator—likely the trigger for a nearby IED to cause more carnage. In less than five minutes, little children would spill into the street, but we had not yet heard back from our commanding officer. We didn't have permission to engage and were all rendered impotent without permission from on high.

Anxious, our Recon sniper left his rifle and got on the radio to say that we would have a lot of dead children on our hands if we did not get the order immediately. There was no more time left to deliberate. The sniper turned and moved away, radio in hand, while his spotter was trying to add confirmation of the situation. Surely the Command understood what was at stake if we did not act RIGHT NOW with deadly force. Standing next to his rifle, I was ready: binoculars up. I watched the school door fly open just as the insurgent aimed his weapon.

There's no time!

Our sniper wasn't in position, so I instantly dropped to the ground, visualized the target, and fired. The shot hit the target's mid- to upper-back, and though he was down, I was too late. He got a shot off but was not able to reach the detonator. As our sniper rushed over to his weapon, I was still, until my perspective shifted. Far above everything, I could see clearly through the confusion.

I had committed a war crime since I was a doctor, who was not supposed to be involved in active combat; I also did not have permission to fire from the Command. I was not quick enough in my disobedience. I didn't stop a child from being shot. A child was already injured, maybe killed, but the bomb had not been detonated. The entire situation was wrong.

The Recon sniper pushed me out of the way, assessing the land for further threats while his spotter was cussing at me, furious that they did not get the kill. The gunny (enlisted Marine in charge of the mission) pulled me aside to ask an entirely appropriate question:

"Of the people, by the people, for the people" - Abraham Lincoln

"What the fuck did you do, Doc?"

I had no time for questions or answers. There were two people with bullet wounds in need of my help—a child and the adult enemy combatant who shot her, who had been shot by me.

By the time we made it to the location, the enemy combatant and the child he shot were next to each other. The child's injuries were not life-threatening; there was, however, a through-and-through bullet wound to her lower leg. She was in pain, but a tourniquet would do.

Thirty seconds to stabilize. A lifetime to recover.

For now, she only needed minor interventions, while the enemy soldier's chest wound would require far more work.

His injuries take priority...but where's the justice in that?

Who am I fighting? Is it really up to me to decide who lives and who dies?

If justice is even a concept in war, who would be better treated?

An innocent child or the man who shot her?

In this situation, the one innocent party was a child, paying for everyone else's mistakes.

*****

Then I woke up.

None of it had happened.

It was only a dream, very loosely based on reality.

I didn't kill anyone in Iraq, and though I came close a couple of times during the combat deployments, ultimately, I was preoccupied with my work as a doctor, not as a military officer. Even after thirteen years, these nightmares keep returning. There's one continuous theme: I'm placed in peril, although there's no right path forward. I'm pressed. I need to do something that I am neither qualified for nor prepared to carry out. It's my lot, though. Decide...or make the whole thing worse. Time is limited. Kill one or another will die. Save one and sacrifice one. These assessments are not trivial. They are verdicts that demand instant adjudication without any deliberation or counsel from others.

The nightmares throw me into contorted, life-and-death battles, which is not of my choosing or design. I'm singled out as judge, jury and executioner. Even worse, almost every decision involves switching roles from one moment to the next, each with its singular, core mission. As a military officer, I learned that, often, "the best medicine is to put lead downfield." However, when the dreamy violence is over, I'm thrust into a doctor's work again, healing everyone as if I were in a cartoon with a line of Wile E. Coyotes, all patched up and perfectly healthy (in the frames immediately following a catastrophic injury).

Even though these different "hats" once seemed to produce an incongruent persona, over time, I realized that I was the same person, regardless of the activity. I was still a military officer, performing surgery, just as much as I was a doctor while carrying out military duties.

Time can allow one's perspective to flourish; our memories are not as sharp and, therefore, not as threatening. Over time, I, along with most veterans, came to understand that we never fought an enemy in a different uniform. The only enemy is the human condition. And, since we all are the vessel within which

"Of the people, by the people, for the people" - Abraham Lincoln

the human condition exists, we are left fighting ourselves—the image of God, captured in another (if you are religious). Ultimately, we were at war with vulnerabilities that transcend religious constructs or political power-plays. It's a bitter pill because often, no one is *more right*. So, when we are intolerant of foreign cultures, societal mores, and lifestyles, it's far easier to choose conflict, to destroy the opposing point of view rather than to embrace our shared humanity, and to love one another with our actions.

The thing about the human condition is that it is always present. While new circumstances may bring out different facets of our nature, the truth remains. We start wars because of prejudice and idiocy that could probably be resolved peacefully (if all parties involved would sit down with a good therapist and held themselves to a higher ideal than what they espouse as immutable truth). Hate is also part of the human condition, and like a rabid dog, its evil must be eradicated. Because, when it can propagate, especially within religious extremes or political constructs, it can take on its own life and wage an unnecessary war, producing unhealthy outcomes like generational hatred, genocide, and a collapse of a system. Fear is also ever present, whispering in our ear to protect ourselves and "our own" from enemies foreign and domestic. Unfortunately, fear can be ubiquitous in almost any situation in life and it is an emotion that clouds potential, puts blinders on perspective, and prevents magnanimous thoughts and actions. Fear in war is an obvious daily ritual. It permeates everything, becoming the new norm so much that it is no longer even perceived as fear anymore. It is just how it is. Fear in politics produces a situation that we now have in the USA: nobody talking to each other and both sides of the aisle willing to fall on their own ideological sword, instead of gathering around the flag pole and raising it high for the world to see that we are still standing tall, proud, and free.

Prejudice, idiocy, hate and fear are not a good recipe for anything healthful, and the longer you see the world through these glasses, the more it seems natural and normal. And the more anything seems natural and normal, the harder it is to break free of its mold, as once mindsets have been cast they seem predestined to remain shackled and stagnant. The health care debate, much like the debate on what wars are justified, is rife with emotion and circumstance and this is one of the reasons why the debate on both of these topics seems timeless. For health care, people tend to respond to any discussion on the topic from a foundation of prejudice, idiocy, hate or fear, and then the discussion is aborted before it has been given a chance to construct viable options. We seem to bury the above emotions in nonsensical circular statements that are not meant to stimulate constructive thought. Instead, they are emotional statements (not questions) based out of prejudice, idiocy, hate or fear, which naturally lead to unsubstantial responses:

If everyone had health care would I still get the same quality of care that I have now?

Who's going to pay for it?

Is there enough to go around?

Would I lose the ability to choose my own doctor like I did with the ACA?

"Of the people, by the people, for the people" - Abraham Lincoln

Would there be scarcity rather than abundance with universal health care?

There is nothing wrong with the above questions and they are important questions, because if health care is not done right, the answers to the above will be catastrophically important. The system we have now is so close to failure that any reactionary, fearful, or poorly executed plan could topple it. The problem is not in the questions, the problem is that we do not ask the questions sincerely as we have lost the art form of asking a question and then listening to a thoughtful response. Instead of asking questions with a genuine curiosity, listening and then processing the answer, we ask questions from a dogmatic foundation of prejudice, idiocy, hate or fear.

Just like me reacting to the situation in the dream by pulling the trigger on another human, when we start the health care debate from a position of prejudice, idiocy, hate or fear we are then relegated to reactionary thoughts and policies that have mortal consequences. The questions need to be asked as they, and many others, are vitally essential to move forward in a cohesive and comprehensive manner. But we must be willing to listen.

In health care and in war, ideals are not meant to outweigh the value of human life. That scale cannot be balanced. It is time that we approach the debate with a new perspective and start asking better questions, from a broad hopeful perspective, like:

What would human potential look like if everyone had access to health care, education, good nutrition, and adequate housing?

How would corporations become more profitable if the "unknown cost" of health care for their employees was reasonable and predictable?

"Of the people, by the people, for the people" - Abraham Lincoln

What would society look like if everyone were as healthy as pos-sible and took personal responsibility for their own health as well as the country's health?

How will we pay for the system while balancing the need for health care for all with the need to be fiscally sound and sustain-able, while delivering great quality of care?

Ask a better question from an expansive and inclusive point of view and get a better answer. Ask to listen, not to try to find the loophole in the other person's thoughts so you can then pounce on them, belittle their point of view, and wholeheartedly miss an opportunity to connect and understand.

*****

During my second deployment, I taught World Religions and Introduction to Biology to members of Recon BN for college credit. A handful of the Marines and sailors took advantage of this offering and took one or both courses. During the World Religions course, every person came to the same conclusion on their own: in the eyes of the Iraqis, we were fighting a religious war. Once they understood our Judeo-Christian heritage and the Islamic traditions, they saw as clear as day that we were defend-ing the religion of the USA. President George W. Bush admitted as much in a few of his speeches when he said that our freedoms and "way of life" were being threatened by Saddam Hussein. But this "way of life" is antithetical to those in the Islamic tradition. For them, the USA's culture and democratic governance is syn-onymous with Christianity, and while we may not understand this since we live in a free nation that strives for the separation of church and state, it is blatantly obvious to the Iraqis. They're willing to die with zeal for their religion, which means fight us to the death when we try to free them from an oppressive regime. Unfortunately, in their culture, democracy and unfettered consumerism and Christianity are synonymous; conversely, America's perception of a deplorable, totalitarian regime with rampant civil rights violations also has a name: Islam. I doubt either religion is terribly happy with these associations, yet, they both preach their support for health, love, family, dreams, happiness, and security. Why can't we understand and value one another when we all agree on what's worthy in the world? The same is true for the debate on health care; indeed, there must be goals and measurable outcomes that we can all agree upon as practical people instead of going to war with each other over details that are not immutable truths.

For the health care debate, it seems more fruitful to start at the point where we reach agreement: every member of a society should be as healthy as possible. Then we ask good questions: how do we get there? And what are the consequences, wanted and unintended, of achieving this lofty goal? To carry out substantive and inclusive health care reform, we must align ourselves with both sides of the story without wholesale support of a political party's ideology (which should **NEVER** be confused with a belief system like a "way of life." There is a very good reason our forefathers put separation of church and state in our Constitution and we would be wise to remember their creed). In Iraq, I wrestled with who I was supposed to be—a doctor or an officer?

"Of the people, by the people, for the people" - Abraham Lincoln

Now, it's evident that I was both at the same time, and while that produced some natural cognitive dissonance, making it difficult to feel "whole," I needed to grasp how I am defined by more than just one or two things. When it comes to health care policy and debate, I promise that you are more than only a Republican or a Democrat or a welder or a nurse or a part-time pastry chef. You are multiple personas mixed into the wonderfulness that is you, and if you hold on to all the components of your identity (even the contradictions), then you will have a better chance of finding common ground with those who oppose your point of view, instead of crashing into an impasse. Prejudice, idiocy, hate and fear do not belong in this debate, and it is time that we honestly come to the table with common goals and see where the conversation takes us. Political parties are NOT a belief system and should not be followed with the zeal of religious worship. This zeal, this epistemology, this worship belongs to God, not to political agendas and certainly not to debates about things like health care. Have passion, have an educated point of view, but do not have your identity so wrapped up in it that you are willing to go to war with anyone who disagrees. Religion is meant to guide us. Politics is meant to represent the will of the people. When the streams cross between these very different and divergent constructs, devastating results happen whose ripples are felt for centuries to come. (The Crusades, the genocides, the needless wars... Unfortunately, there are too many examples to list.)

But, that's not what we usually do. We as a country are starting to take our thoughts on topics like health care and make them so personal that they need to be defended with religious zeal. We turn away from the myriad concerns of others, we compartmentalize our priorities, and then we shut down all substantive debate. We act as if Moses wrote down what is supposed to happen with health care on one of the stones, directly from the mouth of God. We reject difficult topics while polarizing issues that were never political in the first place. We complain about walls and then wonder about who put the bricks in our hands. We keep building anyway, and the resolution becomes impossible. Unwanted. After this, we want to deconstruct the debate, invalidating the argument, but we also deconstruct the person defending the opposite side. We dismiss them as ill-informed, dumb, a bigot, a sexist, xenophobic. All these labels do is separate us further while we turn away from our true religion, which is fairly explicit that this is not how we are to treat each other. We do not fight these illusions because they allow us an easy out: stick to a dogmatic stance or defend our inequitable policies. Once we understand a different point of view, we might understand why the other side is fighting against us with religious zeal. Once we understand the opposition, we can find common ground where everyone is heard and considered. But where is the obstinate self-righteousness in that?

In the military, I thought of myself as an officer at times when it was convenient, and then, when it suited me better, I was a doctor. If I needed a scapegoat, an excuse, or just needed some distance from someone, I put on a different "hat" that allowed me to escape. Being a chameleon meant that I was not responsible for anything. Had I just been me—a complicated mix of essential and partially incongruent personas—then I would have

"Of the people, by the people, for the people" - Abraham Lincoln

been a whole soul, capable of handling the intricacies a combat doctor at war with himself must face. Instead, I purposely divided myself, limiting my identity to one thing…minute to minute. Shooting the sniper as an officer first, and then assuming the healer role second, is the perfect example of my very convenient and incongruent persona that kept me from accepting the reality of war and any personal responsibility I had for any given situation.

The truth is that, in the dream, I shot the person as Reagan B. Anderson, not as a combat doctor and not as a military officer. I was both of those things, and many more, but neither one defined me. What defined me, even though I was actively rebelling against it at this point in my life, was that I was a child of God doing the very best I could in a very difficult situation. The essential miseries and contradictions faced were not the point. The point was to find a way out of the chaos that was in alignment with who I was, what I was put on this earth to do, and to gain a wisdom that will instruct the future. I was not a religious zealot in a holy war.

How did I get past this pattern of convenient compartmentalization and into the realm of reality, empowering health and wisdom to flourish? How do you approach a tough situation or problem as a whole individual, with a singular mindset—instead of picking one of the thousands of characterizations you've gathered over your lifetime? How do we avoid the seduction of inactivity that is fueled by obstinate prejudice, idiocy, hate and fear? How do we get past the confusion, lack of faith, perception of scarcity, lack of self-confidence, preoccupation with career, conflicting personas?

"Of the people, by the people, for the people" - Abraham Lincoln

Many of us look at a task and say that there is just no way that we could do it on our own. We don't have the resources, the education, the contacts, the time, the marketing—still, we all have accomplished things that defy reason or our resources. If you looked at all of the tasks that you have accomplished, in their totality, most would ask how you did everything. Yet, how many of us have finished a degree? How many of us are parents? How many of us have a finished project that took years to complete? We all have examples of daunting tasks that we have finished and overcome with the simple decision to do so, regardless of cost, while ignoring our excuses. One foot in front of the other completes a worthwhile journey fueled with strength and stamina. Soon, the degree is hanging on the wall, your child is 18 and out of the house, or your project is complete (and done well).

One of the huge lessons that I learned in Iraq was that we, the USA, should not be liberating a people who have not asked for our help. They need to do it for themselves so that they do it the "right" way, taking into consideration their own culture, ideals, and perspectives. If we do it for them, the likely result will be what happened in Iraq and why Iraq still is not a stable country capable of successful self-governance. We do not have the power AND the authority to do this for another country. Wars are poor chisels to bring about peace.

And there are lessons to be learned from this as it relates to the use of our military, as well as the government in the delivery of health care. The government can't in and of itself make this great country healthy. That is up to us, the people. While laws and regulations are important and absolutely must be addressed

"Of the people, by the people, for the people" - Abraham Lincoln

in an intelligent and comprehensive manner, it is ultimately up to us, you and me individually, to make it happen. One thing is certain though, if we go to war with each other over the health care debate, a peaceful and healthful tomorrow will not be created.

WHERE TO START

Health care needs a degree of deconstruction, modernization, and renewal, but revolutions hold daunting work and the "task" probably seems insurmountable to many.

Who knows where we even start to tackle a problem this big?

If we can come to the table as whole individuals, committed to making the healthiest society in history, while focusing on shared goals, without approaching it with the religious zeal prescribed by a political party, then we will have the courage it takes to create meaningful, substantive, comprehensive, and sustainable change. While health care is not partisan, it is intensely personal and asks that we embrace our actions and morals, independent of a particular political party's stance. It takes a lot of dedicated, intelligent, compassionate and caring individuals, who will acknowledge their part in the problem, to craft long-lasting solutions. Just like everything else that you have accomplished in life it might seem like an insurmountable task, but that just means that it is worthwhile work and the reward will be well worth the toil. Together we can!

*****

Memorial Day is set aside to celebrate the fallen heroes of our great country and to acknowledge the ultimate sacrifice they

"Of the people, by the people, for the people" - Abraham Lincoln

made so that we can enjoy the freedoms this country affords. Memorial Day for me this year started with the horrible dream in this chapter. Thank God it was just a dream. But I did not tell you about the rest of my day—it was glorious. The sun was shining, the air was inviting, my wife was beautiful, and I was safe, surrounded by friends and family over a barbecue overlooking Pikes Peak, the mountain that inspired "America the Beautiful." I was overcome with gratitude that I was free to build my life how I saw fit in the land of the free, home of the brave. It is an amazing privilege and one I hope to never stop appreciating. Even though Memorial Day is a hard day for me, because too many men and women have died for this great country, this year it was full of grace and peace. Even though Iraq was difficult, it has given me a perspective that is invaluable. The road to health after Iraq was a long one that started with a commitment to once again be healthy and to start fulfilling my life's work. It was a journey of a thousand miles but the destination was well worth the steps. One day, I will look back on the long journey it has taken this country, individually and collectively, to get to a good health care system that works for everyone, and it too will be worth it. I understand the work ahead will not be easy but I also know that now is the time, today is the day, and you and I are the resources that are needed to complete this journey.

It starts with just one step,
together,
in the land of the free,
home of the brave.

"Of the people, by the people, for the people" - Abraham Lincoln

AFTER ACTION REVIEW:

- Today, ask yourself what emotional, spiritual, and political attachment you have to the health care debate. Actually, take a moment to understand the basis of your thoughts on health care and then write them down below so that they are out in the open, ready to be scrutinized by you.

- Put yourself in the shoes of someone who does not have adequate health care for themselves or their loved ones and ask what emotional, spiritual, and political attachments they have to the health care debate. Write down how you think they come to the ballot box and what is important to them.

"Of the people, by the people, for the people" - Abraham Lincoln

NOTES:

NOTES:

Chapter 8

AmeriCAN or AmeriCAN'T?

"Some blunders and absurdities no doubt crept in; forget them as soon as you can. Tomorrow is a new day.

You shall begin it serenely and with too high a spirit to be encumbered with your old nonsense."
-Ralph Waldo Emerson

WHY WRITE A BOOK like this, and why read it? Why divulge failures and immaturities within unpleasant discussions of war? Why detail embarrassingly essential missteps in my vocational and personal lives? Why would I invite you to see the warts and wrinkles of a dermatologist? They are all great questions. Documentation is also potentially problematic. It invites scrutiny. Who does that? And, as a respected member of the community, why risk being vulnerable?

Vulnerability makes the human condition indomitable.

The answer is at once simple and very complex for an individual, an ideology, a society, because it starts with an honest and maybe painful self-examination and willingness to be open/vulnerable to another person's ideas and perceptions.

Before we can have a constructive dialogue with anyone else, we must first understand our own perceptions, and to do that we must be willing to look at our experiences, our successes, our failures, our prejudices and our beliefs, and from that try to really understand ourselves. Being self-aware requires honesty and the willingness to lower our defensive shields, take off our "game face," become vulnerable, and from that become stronger because we have then stripped away—or at least become aware of—the ties that bind us to past negative or counterproductive ideas that can stand in the way of progress for ourselves or, by extension, for the society in which we live. So why explore these things that can be uncomfortable? Because it's the first step in a many-step process leading to the final, rational, nonpolitical realization that while people may disagree on the road map, we might agree on the ultimate destination. If we can agree on the ultimate destination then we are one step closer to acknowledging that there is more than one way to get there. If we can accept that, then perhaps we can also (maybe grudgingly) accept that just because another person's side/religion/political affiliation is different from ours, he or she might actually have something intelligent to say and we might actually have more in common than not. If we can accept that, which requires that we have enough self-awareness and humility to also accept that perhaps our own perspective could use some fine-tuning, then we are on the road to meaningful dialogue. If we can actually have an open and honest dialogue, then we have a chance at agreement or at least "peaceful coexistence" that allows us as a society to arrive at our mutual destination.

"Of the people, by the people, for the people" - Abraham Lincoln

And all of this starts with us being honest. We need to start being honest about who we are and how we arrived here. That includes the good, the bad, and the necessary uncomfortable experiences that have given us the wisdom to change the world. All of it needs to be brought to life—honestly and genuinely—which, in turn, creates a new cycle. Our assertions of the past will free others, encouraging them to admit their failings and celebrate their successes. We reach our most powerful peak when we are sincere about who we are and what we have learned. This process can gain momentum, and then strength translates to an informed society privileged to live its passions and chase its dreams with abundant health and vitality.

So, why write this book and why read it? Because we as a society are being smothered by lies, "spin," and irrational emotion all based on fear, greed, ego, which leads to polarization which then leads to paralysis and can lead to rebellion. If this continues, we are in danger of dousing the spark that has made our country the envy of the world and before that, watching our health care system disintegrate.

I hope that the stories and messages of this book encourage you to seek out the company of others who do not necessarily believe as you do. If we can become self-aware enough to understand our own motivations and needs and ideas, respect that others have equally strong motivations, needs, ideas with identities, and that disagreement does not equal "right" and "wrong," then we can achieve a society full of divergent opinions—all pointing in the same, healthful direction.

Once we can accept that disagreement doesn't equal right,

"Of the people, by the people, for the people" - Abraham Lincoln

and start having an honest dialogue with ourselves and with others, we will have a fruitful path forward. We live in a day and age in which many of us manufacture our image on social media, disregarding the beautifully complex narrative that makes us. One is tempted to start believing that everyone else wakes up and marches off into their perfect worlds. Everything is in its right place. And meanwhile, you're over here—thinking you're a mess, consuming what's comfortable—when the truth is that you're a kaleidoscope of successes and failures, experiences wanted and not, thoughts shared and reserved. We've all made mistakes; it's not just you. I hope my story is a polemic for raw, painful truths, and rails against manufactured pretenses. That's uncomfortable and at times perhaps sad. Yet, it also shows the triumph and indomitability of the human spirit.

I have witnessed a profound shift in societal wisdom after forty-five years of walking this planet. Growing up, I remember the older generations having strength and wisdom that came from honest dialogue and curiosity into what made others tick. My father and his father debated events, trying to create a more cohesive perspective towards political and societal equanimity. While at times these debates would get heated, they never crossed the line of disrespect, character judgment, or hostility. And, what's more, they both looked forward to the discussions and looked forward to what the other could teach. When Granddad would visit, the whole family knew the schedule. Immediately following dinner, politics were discussed until 2:00 or 3:00 AM when my stepmother would wake up and tell the men that they needed to sleep. They did (reluctantly like two kids who did not want to miss the party by going to sleep), but they had a new understanding that would have remained undiscovered had they not taken the time to listen to each other from a position of openness, confidence, strength, and vulnerability.

Today, we discourage that same brand of healthy and instructive discourse. We've lost our curiosity and analytical thinking. Plus, it's hard to connect when everyone you know is trying to manufacture a persona unmoored from vulnerable reality. False personas are fragile because they can't carry their weight. They can't defend themselves. And it is this weakness that feeds the need to rehearse conspiracies, endorse unsound arguments, and to insult those with opposing viewpoints. However, what they lack in cohesive thought, they make up for in ruthlessness. They expose their ignorance through personal attacks and a cold, indignant and self-righteous refusal to communicate. Though there are at least two sides to the dispute, one or both sides shut themselves off to reason, choosing to invalidate the opposition's argument and their person if at all possible. Instead of looking for real connection, they imagine sordid relationships, jump on buzzwords, and endeavor to trap their opponents. Anyone with a conflicting opinion has a brand: *stupid, bigot, communist, or...* that makes it easier to dismiss. Instead of searching for understanding, they take the self-righteous path, and cut off the argument, calling others "horrible people," and spouting that the only salvation is for others to shut up and agree with their own omniscient and infallible stance. There is absolutely no room for honest, valuable discussion with that kind of weakness. Weakness begets intolerance, which is then manifested by what the media vomits onto its audience and what we see play out in social media. We become increasingly polarized into tribes of "true believers."

For instance, there is the contentious subject of gun control in America. When was the last time you heard someone on the opposite side of the issue say something to this effect:

"I so appreciate your having a dialogue with me, since we both want the same thing for the USA: safety and security. While your idea on how to do that differs from mine, we still have a common goal! I'm sure that, in time, we will find a mutually agreeable solution if we keep focusing on safety and security. So, please tell me how you think we should make the USA safe and secure regarding the topic of gun control."

Imagine hearing that on the news! You would think that it was a *Saturday Night Live* skit in which a resurrected John Belushi is about to crash through a wall dressed as a samurai. Unfortunately, today, we're more likely to see a reiteration of the old *Saturday Night Live* skit in which Dan Ackroyd responds to a solid argument with, "Jane, you ignorant slut!" This comment, which was funny thirty years ago due to its preposterous nature, would not be considered so in the present. Very unfortunately, it is now the new norm for our "news."

Our tolerance for polarization perpetuates a toxic political climate in which power is wielded by the obstinate and judgmental and therefore kept away from the people. It is deliberate, and it works. Democracy is being taken hostage and it is time that we the people take it back by being willing to shed our political affiliations and start actively participating in the dialogue.

"Of the people, by the people, for the people" - Abraham Lincoln

The only answer to the societal degradation infecting our great country is to have a free dialogue about our thinking, our behavior, and our betrayals. We need to understand how our perspectives shifted and identify ways to persevere in the face of human fallibility.

I hope that the stories and messages of this book encourage you to seek out the company of others who do not necessarily believe as you do. If we can become comfortable with identities and abilities in the face of pain, then we will achieve a society full of divergent opinions—all pointing in the same, healthful direction.

I also intend to encourage a dialogue about peace, nonviolence, and war, as I empathize with each position. I started this journey in seminary, through the lens of epistemology, where I encountered a peaceful, sensible world. Now, I think that reason dictates the times and situations (although admittedly few and far between) in which the only answer is to violently murder evil, swiftly and without remorse. My ideological shift was not intentional. It was an obligation forged out of horrendous experiences. I have tried to explain what transpired, what ripped a warm and comfortable worldview to shreds, and what could replace it at times: a coldly swinging guillotine. Now, I'm not advocating for such a "black and white" worldview in which there is only room for either nonviolence or for "crying havoc," as that would be wholly inappropriate and each represents only one side of the coin. Instead, I believe the world would be better if we all understood the nonviolent as well as the violent approach so that wisdom may prevail for which one to use, when to use

"Of the people, by the people, for the people" - Abraham Lincoln

it, and when to go to the other side of the coin. My hope is that war is as sickening for you as it is for me, and that same horror will steer your future decisions with an intellectual knowledge of war—minus the price required to attain it. In my opinion, no one should have the power to resolve military conflict unless he or she can intrinsically and viscerally appreciate the nuanced and inevitable consequences of this type of violence. Hopefully, reading the stories in this book will provide another way for you to consider nonviolence as well as violence, eschewing self-righteous positions for empathetic ones.

In many of our debates, we as a society do agree. Even in the gun debate, we agree. We want safety, physical and economic security, and good health. Both sides want this. We agree! We just have perhaps radically disparate beliefs on how we will achieve those things. We want our fellow Americans to find happiness, to strive to be better, and to be free, although the maps we use to get there are wild and conflicting. The debate about universal health care is equally contentious; but again, we agree on what we all want: to be healthy. Yet, we gorge on misinformation that feeds our fears, not accurate knowledge that motivates our ingenuity. Enough is enough.

I was inspired to write after studying health care delivery with a Master of Public Health, after delivering care to those under my medical privilege in radically different environments, and after looking into the abhorrent VA system. As a doctor with seventeen years of experience at war and in peace; as a teacher for the next generation of dermatologists; as an author of textbook chapters, published articles, this book; as a national health

"Of the people, by the people, for the people" - Abraham Lincoln

care lecturer; as a member of the board at a national health care college; and as an owner of a private practice for over nine years, I am ready to throw all of me in the ring to fight for common sense in the health care debate. Like most things in life, the more you know, the more questions you have. With that being said, I do think the wealth of evidence points in one general nuanced direction with some important factors needing to be taken into consideration. I also believe that once fears are addressed honestly and with honor, we might just have a different perspective on the topic of universal health care.

As a former combat doctor and current physician treating many active and retired military and their dependents, I believe any discussion of the USA's health care system must include the medical services provided by the Veterans Administration, supposedly designed to uphold the promise made to everyone who joins the military that they will receive lifetime medical care for injuries sustained in the service of this great country. As it turns out, the VA is the poster boy of broken promises and bureaucratic bungling at its worst (more on this in Section 3 of this book). The military has always been used as pawns by the elected elite, those born into privilege, and those who cannot appreciate the struggle. They do not know what it tastes like—to hunt and be hunted. During a war, both sides of the political aisle smack their lips, spinning the blood, sweat, and tears of our warriors into political currency. Then, when the war is over, they pivot, deciding on how to exploit us for their next election. Very few of them care, which is palpable each time Congress investigates the VA. In its present form, it's a disgrace, but that would not be the case if only a few of our politicians made an effort to organize the care for our veterans. There are a few champions of the military and I celebrate them: the late Senator John McCain, who is one of the true heroes of my lifetime; Congressman Doug Lamborn, who does so much behind the scenes that we all owe him our respect and appreciation; and a handful of others who seem to care more about the military than anything they stand to gain politically. I salute those who are honestly trying to help our veterans.

When politicians play up public support for our veterans, without any movement behind the scenes, generational distrust of our government is created among the warriors in our society. I'd urge caution; if this abuse goes on long enough, the spirit that founded the USA will feel compelled to remake itself through another revolution by the people, for the people, and of the people. Right now, this revolution can start with us demanding more of our politicians, the media, and ourselves. Instead of encouraging the power-hungry policies of hate and discontent that keep citizens powerless and in the dark, now is the time to rise up, lead by example, and approach topics like health care from a position of openness and strength. Only then will we take back the power that has been stripped from us. For the power in a democracy rests on the shoulders of its citizens. The power of a dictatorship rests on the shoulders of the elite, and I doubt many of us are happy with the power dynamics in the USA right now.

*****

"Of the people, by the people, for the people" - Abraham Lincoln

I humbly and vulnerably write, inviting you into the joy, sorrow, triumph, and disaster of my life's journey (so far). Now, the stories of war are over and I hope that you have come away from the first section of the book with a couple of thoughts:

- The health care debate is not a partisan issue. It is about health, not disingenuous political pandering.
- We all have different experiences in life that have given us strength and the perspective to back up our thoughts and opinions. It is time we start listening to others as we all want the same things in life. It is time we start taking ownership of the problem, get educated, get involved, and take back the power that is rightfully ours—the citizens of this great country.
- Our "health care" system is about to fracture and we need true leadership to navigate through the rough waters.

It's impossible for me to see where you are, what you have been through, or what you are striving toward in your life. Still, I hope that these stories and discussions will provide you with a personal touchstone—something new to consider—and perhaps, a brighter direction. We are a part of the greatest country ever, and to whom much is given, much will be expected. May we be proud of the rule of law and the examples that we leave, because when we lead, the world follows. May we do it well, from a position of emotional depth, strength, vulnerability, and of course, gratitude.

The rest of the book is an attempt to give you, the reader, my thoughts on how to move forward with the debate on health care with specific recommendations and ideas to consider. Each idea

"Of the people, by the people, for the people" - Abraham Lincoln

is born out of a desire to bring greater health to our country and to secure a fiscally responsible and abundantly healthy future that will last for generations to come. They are just my thoughts though, and they will need modification as the evidence emerges and as different perspectives illuminate problems with my theories. And, I am more than okay with that. Collective intelligence is better than individual intelligence = the foundation of democracy. Let's agree to first consider my opinions, then to individually evaluate them based on your own research, experiences and wisdom, as well as how other countries have implemented their health care systems with a discerning eye to what could and what could not work for the USA; then agree to come to the table with how to make everything better in an open, honest, and honoring dialogue.

My father has taught me from an early age that he does not care to hear what he can't do. He has no time for "can't." He wants to know what he "CAN" do. Likewise, as we approach the rest of the book let's get rid of the "can't" mentality that will stifle any chance for progress. The media and our politicians are infamous for telling us what we can't do because it gives them all the power. The tyranny of "can't" is called a dictatorship. The freedom of "CAN" is called democracy of the people, by the people, and for the people. Let's figure out what we "CAN" do and then do it! The very future of our democracy depends on it.

Together, we CAN!!!
Together, we MUST!!!
Together, we WILL!!!

"Of the people, by the people, for the people" - Abraham Lincoln

AFTER ACTION REVIEW:

- Ask yourself, what are the fundamental ingredients that make a democracy work and then ask yourself for whom the current system is working, who has the power, and how that has affected your day-to-day life. Write down your thoughts below on what examples the media and our politicians are setting and what you think the natural course of their actions will produce for your children, and your children's children.

- Then, write down what the country would look like if we took back the power of "can't" from those who have bought into this philosophy.

- Finally, write down two major personal life stories, and ask yourself what leadership/wisdom/perspective these experiences have given you and how they will help you get involved with being an AmeriCAN.

"Of the people, by the people, for the people" - Abraham Lincoln

NOTES:

NOTES:

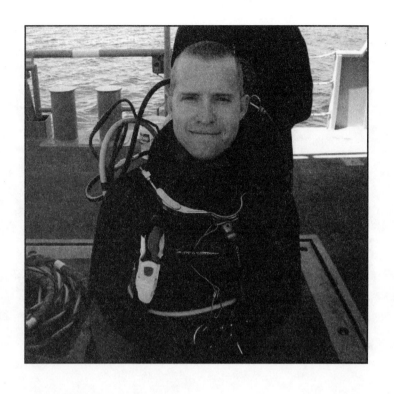

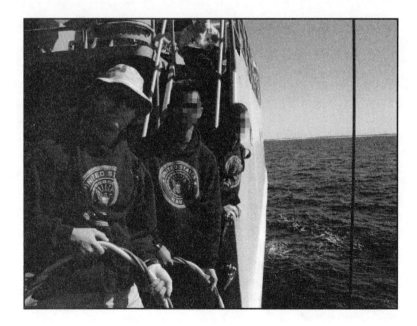

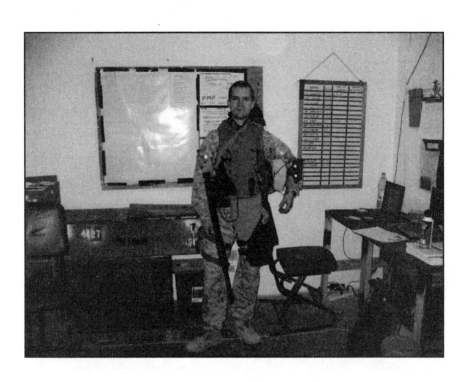

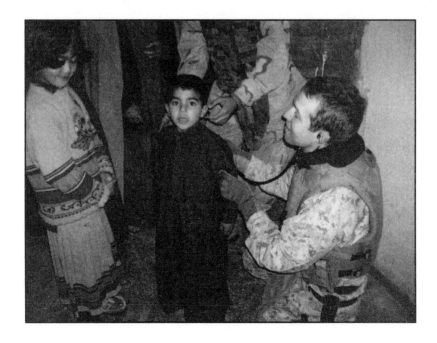

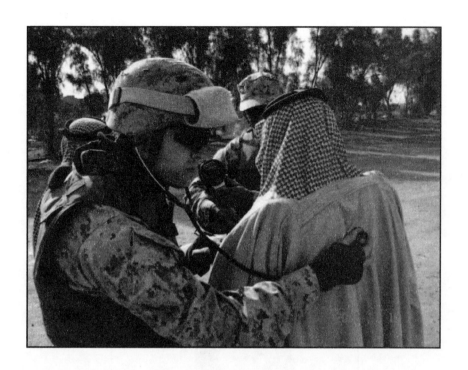

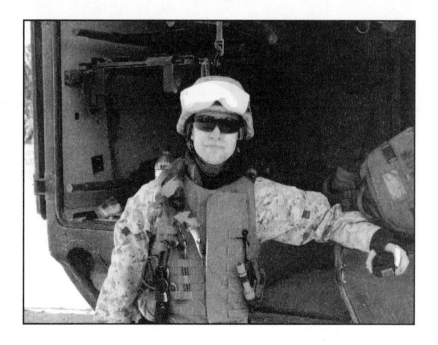

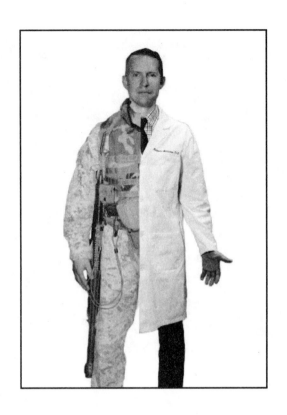

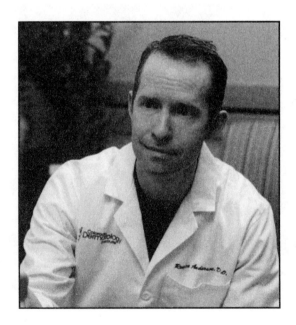

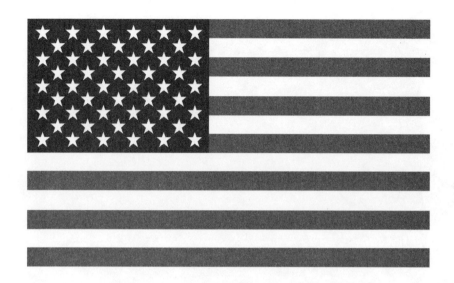

SECTION II

CHAPTER 9

BURNT OUT

"How the fuck am I supposed to do good medicine on fifty patients a day? Plus rounds? ... I fight over billing. I fight over prescription coverage. Insurance companies are dedicated to not paying you. And the big law firms, man. They are just waiting. They're just betting that you are going to make that one big mistake. This profession, for me, was a higher calling. You know, make people's lives better."
-Drunk Doctor Stan's rant from *Love and Other Drugs*

PHYSICIANS BURN OUT at an alarming rate, between 32 and 68% depending on their specialty! Physicians have among the highest, if not the highest, suicide rates of any profession. Physicians are at the end of their rope. There are many issues that factor into this, and the argument of this book is that a big portion of our health care problems in the USA stems from it being more "death care" amongst the entitled instead of health care for the accountable. While the causes are many, malpractice plays a significant role in these statistics, and that is the focus of this chapter. It is a huge issue that probably affects you more than it does the medical providers who have a target on their backs.

A friend of mine, who's been practicing for fifteen years, has been sued three times. He didn't have to settle the lawsuits because he did nothing wrong. They were frivolous, but lawyers took the cases, drawn by potentially massive settlements. He won all of them, yes, but the emotional damage it deals is catastrophic for a physician's professional and private lives. The consequence of being sued is the temptation to practice "defensive medicine," to be more burnt out, to think that patients are not partners but instead are potential adversaries. The price of "defensive medicine" (to protect against frivolous, unfounded litigation) is estimated to be at least $46 billion annually in the USA as providers order more tests, more consults, more of everything to try to protect themselves as much as possible![3] But we know the actual cost is mountains more than just a financial hit to you and to the system.

I view patients as partners, aiming for a common goal. I entered the field because, like our doctor's quotation above, it is a higher calling. Still, I had no idea what practicing medicine in the USA was like. I couldn't anticipate the dangers I'd be fighting every day, and I certainly did not foresee the obstacles specifically designed to deny access to care so that the big business behind the "system" could be more profitable. It was simpler in my mind: I imagined educating patients about how to stay healthy, and followed by their compliance, we would adjust course as necessary throughout their lifetime. Nothing could be more untrue.

---

3 Mello MM, Chandra A, Gawande AA, Studdert DM. National costs of the medical liability system. Health affairs. 2010 Sep;29(9):1569–1577.

"Of the people, by the people, for the people" - Abraham Lincoln

Prevention is not part of treatment, so it's not taught in public, private, undergraduate, or medical school; prevention doesn't make money, so it is not encouraged by any part of the system. I was trained at the founding school of osteopathic medicine. Osteopathic physicians are supposed to be holistic practitioners. If any doctor is supposed to know about prevention, it is the osteopathic physician. However, we had less than forty hours, less than one week out of a grueling four-year curriculum, of education on diet, exercise, and mental wellbeing—the absolute foundation of any healthy life. In residency, there was not even one minute spent learning anything about prevention except to stay out of the sun. In contrast, we spent literally hundreds (if not thousands) of hours learning about prescriptions, even more hours about treatment for things that could have been prevented in the first place, and a lifetime of fighting against a system that has been designed for profit, not health.

If we even had the education to teach preventative medicine, providers get paid less to teach patients about prevention than they do to write a prescription that will just mask the symptoms. Doctors learn how to treat disease, really, once it is too late for health. We don't learn how to prevent it. We're relied upon, valued, and paid when disease is already present. We are intervention, only. We primarily focus on disease and death, not on keeping people healthy. Our business is disease; unfortunately, business is very good at approximately 18% of GDP and expected to be upwards of 25% of GDP in the next twenty years—far and away the most expensive "health care" per capita in the world. To add insult to injury, while we have the most expensive health

"Of the people, by the people, for the people" - Abraham Lincoln

care in the world, we rank near the bottom of health care in the industrialized world in terms of actually keeping people healthy. The parts and participants of the USA's "health care system" have fractured and it is just a matter of time before gangrene sets in.

THE PAST

Before medical school, I lived in Vancouver, Canada and attended college and then an ecumenical seminary, leading services and church youth groups. I walked the alleys of Vancouver feeding drug addicts, sex workers, and the oppressed, and since I had no money, I paid for my room and board with cleaning, nannying and dumpster diving for food. I had dedicated my extra resources to buying food for the hungry and then handing out sandwiches. I know this is highly unusual, and something that I do not recommend as it is very dangerous. I used to think that the only thing people would need to get off the streets was for someone to believe in them, feed them, listen, show them love. I thought that if those needs were met, then they would be free to change their lives for the better. So, two nights per week, I did what I could to help others. A lot of my stories are unbelievable. Some are more like sordid scenes from *Pulp Fiction*.

Heading down an alley around 11:00 PM, I was startled by the abrupt motion of a man, who ripped his shirt open wide, and then fell on his back. I watched as a woman jumped on top of him, raised her hand, and stabbed him in the chest with a needle filled with heroin—after a few seconds, she straightened up to look at me. Then, when the man sat up, I offered them sandwiches.

"Of the people, by the people, for the people" - Abraham Lincoln

He had been "chasing the dragon"—using black tar heroin—for the last five years. It had destroyed every accessible vein and artery in his body. The visible ones were shot, along with the invisible, the easily accessed blood vessels, and even the veins underneath his fingernails were full of scar tissue. He was also missing a couple of fingers due to his addiction. We just sat and talked and ate as if nothing had happened. But at the end of the day, he kept "chasing the dragon," content to not better his situation no matter what everyone around him was trying to do for him.

Because of these experiences, I dreamed of becoming a doctor and serving an inner-city population. I planned to buy a big apartment building and have a medical clinic on the first floor. Tenants would be limited to those who needed help medically and vocationally. I would take care of their medical needs so that they would be healthy, and then I would pay for them to attend a trade school of their choice with the agreement that, after they graduated, their first job would be to practice their trade in their apartment. After that, they'd work on the rest of their apartment complex to improve their home and gain valuable experience. They would purchase their units with thriving wages. Once they had some experience after school, they could apply for local positions, or start a business. After completing the building and converting it to a co-op, then I would relocate to another building—personally owning nothing—as the mission would be of the people, for the people, by the people.

I went to medical school with lofty aspirations of saving the world, one soul at a time. I felt called to the profession and went at it with all the zeal that a "calling" dictates. The first rotation

"Of the people, by the people, for the people" - Abraham Lincoln

of third-year medical school was at an inner-city free clinic in Detroit. I was so excited. While it was not the *exact* dream of delivering health care as I described, it was pretty close. What I found shocked me. Patients came into the clinic to get another Sexually Transmitted Disease (STD) treatment that year instead of behaving in ways that could prevent them (it was not unusual for a patient to have over five STDs in a year); others were picking up narcotics for "chronic pain" when there were no signs that they were actually in pain; healthy men came in, asking for doctor's notes to take the day off work. The list of ridiculous complaints never ended. After one month at the free clinic, it was readily apparent that, for 99 percent of the population, we were doing more harm than good. As providers, we actively perpetuated their state! Few, if any, wanted help to get back on their feet. When the immediate future is all that matters, it only makes sense to take advantage of the system. I had to find a new reason for staying in medicine. I refused to participate in a system that hindered people from standing on their own. I contemplated leaving medical school. At that juncture, however, I could not walk away without significant, lifelong ramifications. Plus, even though the thought of quitting is often enticing and the subject of frivolous daydreams, quitting is not part of my DNA. So I stayed, hoping that a new purpose would become apparent, and I would find a way to work within the raw reality of medicine.

THE PRESENT

I own a dermatology clinic in Colorado and spend my time removing skin cancers from middle-aged and elderly patients.

"Of the people, by the people, for the people" - Abraham Lincoln

In blissful suburbia, I remove cancer after cancer—it's a far cry from Detroit or Iraq. There is a unique art in cutting a cancer from the nose of a patient who is awake and wondering what his face will look like when the healing ends; there is an absolute honesty that comes in these moments when people are afraid, nervous, and vulnerable. I love my patients. For the most part, they are great people who are appreciative of the help, and my work is needed, valued. Still, this is not how I envisioned my life back in those pre-medical school days. To stay in medicine, my "why" had to change.

Quitting was too enticing. In Iraq, during a mission, there was a moment where I was waiting to attend casualties, and I mused that I would like nothing more than to quit it all and become a chef. A line had been crossed. Medicine was no longer something I could stomach. After eleven years of pursuing one goal, I was willing to split. I wanted to live a different life. While the oppressiveness of the situation in Iraq unfolded, my mind sorted through my real options—

Chef. Transient. Architect. Entrepreneur. Dermatologist...

I had once dated a dermatologist who loved her job. She did not deal with a lot of death and dying, and she certainly did not treat trauma in her day-to-day life. I applied, never believing that I'd be accepted into a dermatology residency because they are far too competitive, and I had spent the last four years in the military instead of doing the things necessary to be a strong candidate. Regardless, I was accepted. I went to Detroit to train under one of the giants in the field, Dr. Steven Grekin. He took me under his wing, taught me dermatology, and helped mend the soul of a hypervigilant, out-of-place young man who didn't see where he would fit in a world after war. It took years of rebuilding but I am at peace with my past and my present.

In my practice, nearly all my patients have insurance. In Colorado Springs, at least half of my patients are military, former military, or have a family member who is. Most are over 55, and apart from their skin needs, they do not need much from me. My purpose has shifted to caring for this patient population, as well as my staff. Customer service is paramount, and we want to set the example for how to treat patients, and how we must treat one another. It is a good profession, though its "why" is dissimilar to the one I had in medical school.

THE FUTURE

There is an as-yet unappreciated and unheard calling that stirs in my soul, telling me that I have another purpose (other than being a doctor). It is palpable and present. Yet, I am a doctor for this season. Whatever the future may hold, I will have to redefine my "why" to be relevant, effective, and to help change this world for the better.

REDEFINING MEDICINE'S "WHY"

The doctor from the quotation at the beginning of this chapter is in crisis. Stan went into medicine because it was a "higher calling." Predestined and set up for success, even before he was born, his "why" was clear: he was put on Earth to be a doctor, to help people live a better life. The problem comes with unavoidable, sharp edges—the evolutions in one's character

"Of the people, by the people, for the people" - Abraham Lincoln

must be assimilated into the professional calling or the weight of it will fracture one's identity. In *Love and Other Drugs*, the doctor has not figured out how to reconcile these two opposing states. It's eating him alive. As a culture, we are divided in the business of medicine. We do not understand our role in health, and without definition, a clear purpose remains beyond our reach.

Just like my vocational "why," health care policy and delivery will change as the nation changes, and that is okay—what we have now is not okay; we have not plainly stated or followed our "why," which has led to abuse by all parties. Without proper checks and balances, we are left with a ragged frame...something that is more akin to death care, not health care.

Currently, the system's goal is to make money off an entitled population, deluded in thinking they have no personal responsibility to maintain a healthy lifestyle, or that they are not intelligent enough to research topics on their own health, or that the "system" is just too big for an individual to be able to effect meaningful change. The destructive nature of each side exacerbates the dilemma, and without a proper framework, it cannot support its weight. We must name our priorities, or we will never find them. Further, without a balanced approach, the excessive greed and systemic abuses of the "system" will continue, unchecked.

To craft a solution, we need to draw and define boundaries. So, what is our goal as a nation for health care? Conversely, what is our goal for individuals? How is it structured? How will we pay for it? Is it a fundamental human right? Who should be held

"Of the people, by the people, for the people" - Abraham Lincoln

accountable? How do we, as flawed humans, build comprehensive methods for health care, unfettered by socioeconomic status and other factors while simultaneously stomping out unhealthy behavior? How can we motivate a society?

We must deliberate these questions, but first, we need to define our "why." I would argue that real health care reform has not occurred because:

1)   We do not understand what we believe about health care (who gets it, what they get, how they get it, when they get it, why they need it in the first place, is our priority prevention or treatment).

2)   Nobody has asked informed questions centering around personal, professional, and societal responsibility.

COMMON GROUND

It is important to unite and share a common platform before we start dissenting on how to meet our objectives. We need a base—somewhere we can return to before, during, and after the debate to keep us on track—one that bans ego, political dogmatism, "group think," and partisan pride. Because again, health care is not a partisan issue. In uniting, we can write a mission statement, a rallying cry, and a plan for the inevitable obstacles. We need to start together and end together, focused on our mutual wellbeing, united.

So, let's start with the basics, unite on some tenets, and build up from there. Yes, the devil is in the details but we should be able to agree on the following (in no particular order):

"Of the people, by the people, for the people" - Abraham Lincoln

Tenet 1: Optimal health frees people to secure, on their own terms, life, liberty, and the pursuit of happiness. Without health, our potential—both individually and societally—is blunted.

Yes, I am directly tying our forefathers' words in the Declaration of Independence to the concept of health care reform. Much like our declaring that we did not have a healthy relationship with England, I believe we also have certain inalienable rights that I do not believe our current "health care" system is securing.

Tenet 2: Increasing the health of individuals will lead to a healthier, whole society.

Any system, any organization, any community is made up of its parts. The healthier the parts, the healthier the community. This means that we all have a responsibility to ourselves, and a responsibility to the community, to be as healthy as possible.

Tenet 3: While an individual should not be required to make a specified set of healthful choices, each person should take responsibility for the sum of those choices; at the same time, the group should not be penalized for an individual's decision (such as rationing of care and/or resources).

I have the right to live how I want as long as it does not adversely impact anyone else. I do not have the right to live in a manner that negatively impacts someone else. Most of our laws are built this way. You are not allowed to blare your music at two in the morning if it bothers your neighbors—that is called "disturbing the peace." There are a hundred examples of this. In

"Of the people, by the people, for the people" - Abraham Lincoln

medicine though, you are allowed to be horrendously unhealthy, which negatively impacts society and mandates that healthy individuals pay your share even though they are being responsible. If you want to be unhealthy, that is your right if and only if you pay for your poor health choices, not if you ask others to pay for them. This is of course talking about preventable conditions, not conditions that we have no control over.

Tenet 4: Health care must be just. We need reasonable legal and administrative protections for our providers. We need to advocate for doctors so that they are supported in practicing essential medicine and not the defensive medicine that is also potentially invasive (and costly).

It must work for everyone. No party can unduly benefit by anything that is one-sided, short-term thinking, politically partisan, or overly onerous. We need reasonable legal and administrative protections for our providers. We need to advocate for providers so that they feel substantiated in practicing essential medicine and not the defensive medicine that is also potentially invasive (and costly).

Tenet 5: Every piece of the health care system must be held to account, not just the provider.

Imagine a system in which you are the only person accountable at your home or place of work. How would that play out? We all know that for any situation to be equitable, every party involved needs to be accountable. Right now, the only party accountable in the "health care" system is the provider. This is obviously a problem.

"Of the people, by the people, for the people" - Abraham Lincoln

Tenet 6: One should have abundant access to resources that promote wholesome choices.

People can only be held accountable if they know what they should and should not do. We must let the people know what they need to do to secure health so they can have life, liberty and the pursuit of happiness. Finances and socioeconomic status need not be factors that limit access.

Tenet 7: Disease prevention is the highest priority.

Disease is enormously expensive and is how the whole system is set up right now. Prevention takes time but ultimately has to be the cornerstone of any successful, sustainable, and abundant system.

Tenet 8: Advancements in health care knowledge and delivery should be encouraged, regardless of profitability.

The USA is one of the great pioneers of health care advancements and needs to remain so. Any health policy reform needs to continue to encourage innovation in health care.

Tenet 9: Health care needs to be affordable, accessible, and sustainable.

All of these are intuitively obvious but most of the health policy reform that is brought before Congress only addresses one or two of the three. But all need to be present in order for health to be present.

Tenet 10: Common sense, not overly obtrusive strategy, needs to rule.

"Of the people, by the people, for the people" - Abraham Lincoln

It turns out that the rule of common sense has come to an end and the rule of the media and political parties is alive and well. It is time for the people to start demanding common-sense solutions instead of what we currently have.

Tenet 11: The system cannot tolerate fraud, waste, or the abuse of resources.

When we think of the above, we immediately think of providers committing fraud by devious acts. And while this behavior can't be tolerated, nor can we continue to allow lobbyists and special interest groups to buy laws that favor them instead of what is reasonable. We can't allow insurance companies to deny care just to make an extra buck. We can't continue to allow the emergency department to be exploited for free care instead of for true emergencies. Every part of the system from the patient to the politicians has to be held accountable.

Tenet 12: Public health policy should encourage the entire population—blind to social influences while attentive to educational, regional, and cultural nuances.

Public health policy should be inclusive of all, which means it will be difficult to craft. We know that the healthier the individuals are in a society, the healthier the society is as a whole. So, while it will be difficult work to make sure that health policy is inclusive, the benefit will be enormous.

Tenet 13: We should not sacrifice our rights to implement health care policy.

"Of the people, by the people, for the people" - Abraham Lincoln

We are a free country and must remain so. Any policy can't compromise our freedoms.

Tenet 14: Health care is not a partisan issue, and as such, partisan power-plays have no role in the discussion.

Health care is not a partisan issue. It is an individual and societal issue that affects us all. We can't approach it from a political ideology but instead as individuals who need adequate health care, now and in the future.

Tenet 15: Health care policy in the US needs to be constitutionally sound and supported by every branch of the government.

One of the reasons this country is great and the beacon of light to the world is our foundation, the Constitution, which was written in blood by our forefathers and countless men and women ever since. We cannot violate the foundation of our country, ever.

Tenet 16: Individuals, businesses, and the government should be able to anticipate their health care expenses year after year.

All of us know that one of the biggest challenges we face determining next year's budget is the uncertainty of medical costs. Businesses struggle with being competitive with overseas companies that do not have to worry about this cost, due to universal health care. American companies are at a distinct disadvantage with having to pay this cost and are not able to predict future costs, so it is hard for them to strategize the future. Individuals also can't predict for the next year, which is a big problem for all of us. Over the last fifty years, medical insurance rates have vastly outpaced inflation from year to year and this is projected to continue.

While these concepts are not exhaustive, they can guide the discussion and we can hopefully unite behind them. How the tenets are carried out may reflect in how you see these issues, how you vote, how you address health care professionals, and what you do for your health. They also lead us back to the "why" of public health care policy, as well as our personal responsibility for being healthy.

> *Quite simply, we acknowledge that no relationship, organization, or country can function at an optimal level without health.*
> *Health is a cornerstone of life, liberty and the pursuit of happiness.*

*****

There is a cognitive dissonance with health care. We hate going to doctors' offices or hospitals. We cringe at the thought of addressing our providers face to face, yet we expect them to embody a passionate calling, to be the best. We avoid doctors due to the cost—whether it's time, money, or fear—and often, the benefit does not justify the expense. We hate bad news. We hate paying the copay, then wondering what the final cost of the visit will be (since no one has printed out a handy list for each visit, procedure, medication, or test yet, and these lists are not even reasonably possible for the vast majority of visits). We wonder when mortality will make its claim on our loved ones. We wonder if the system will be able to sustain us when we need it. We are stuck, depending on an unreliable network and obscured by the convoluted mess of insurance. The system is fractured. Like the drunken doctor, we are shocked at how providers are expected to survive with all the pressures of their environment. The reality is that we are sitting beside him, just on the receiving end of the relationship with a lot more to lose than the doctor if the relationship is not a healthy one, if the advice given is not in our best interest, and if the system is set up in such a way to make money instead of health. Do you think that you are actually getting the best care possible if statistically you have a higher chance of seeing a provider who is burnt out rather than fresh (32 to 68%), depressed rather than present, suicidal rather than vibrant (doctors have some of the highest rates of depression and suicide of any profession)? Just how good is the care you are getting under our current system in which the health care providers need a lot of help themselves?

Like the drunk doctor at the beginning of this chapter who is completely burnt out, medicine is a calling for those in the field. Perhaps we need to consider the reason why our healers need healing and what this means for the system.

Physician, heal thyself. Country, heal thyself. Perhaps the two are in balance.

Doctors get into medicine to make the world better. The "why" *was* simple—to make a radical difference in the world.

"Of the people, by the people, for the people" - Abraham Lincoln

After the rigors of medical school and residency though, most doctors start their careers loaded with financial and emotional debt. We're stung by the real experience, by what the practice of medicine actually entails. Disturbingly, taking care of patients is quite effortless compared to what the insurance carriers mandate, what the government demands, and what we fight against each and every day to give good quality health care in a system that supports disease. The flaws are worse than we expected: what doctors are allowed to do has little to nothing to do with what is right for the patient. To be in this position, it takes talent, dedication, and years of hard work, yet we dread the day when a patient will box us in, then sue us for trying to help. The result is expensive, defensive medicine that places every party at a disadvantage. Again, the "why" is about something other than health, and this must change for any meaningful health care reform to have a chance.

MALPRACTICE

In our increasingly litigious society where anyone can sue anyone for most anything, regardless of facts and without penalty for doing so, medical malpractice lawsuits have metastasized into a lawyer's dream and a doctor's nightmare. The ultimate losers are, ironically, patients.

To illustrate, I recently went through a medical malpractice lawsuit and although I was found to have practiced the standard of care and not guilty of any malpractice, the experience brought into sharp focus how grossly warped medical malpractice has become. From the time the lawsuit was started to the two-week

"Of the people, by the people, for the people" - Abraham Lincoln

jury trial, I and members of my staff spent sixteen months compiling records to send to our attorney, going to depositions, taking pictures, and preparing for trial. During the preparations, our attorneys and our medical malpractice insurance company told us they didn't believe the plaintiff had any real case, yet we still had to spend the time to go through the required motions. With every minute spent by our attorneys and opposing council, not to mention the time my staff spent, the money meter kept spinning until the whole thing cost over $500,000 before it was over. And then we get to the personal side of lawsuits.

It is the job of the attorneys on each side to do the best they can to "win" the case for their client. If the facts are on the side of the attorney, then he can use the facts to plead his case. If the facts are not on the side of the attorney, then we get into the seamy side of the law: "spin the words," intentionally misrepresent the facts, try to get the witness to say what you want them to say, or rely on emotional arguments to sway the jury. This is best illustrated by something the poet Carl Sandburg wrote that I understand is something many lawyers learn: "If the facts are against you, argue the law. If the law is against you, argue the facts. If the law and the facts are against you, pound the table and yell like hell." In short, the idea that justice is blind and trials are decided based on merit and truth is, sadly, no more true in medical malpractice cases than it is in many other cases that end up being tried by jury. So, who "won" and who "lost" in this scenario? Well, while I was found "not guilty," which was certainly a relief and a vindication of the many protocols and procedures we've put in place in the clinic to protect patients'

"Of the people, by the people, for the people" - Abraham Lincoln

safety, the real winner was my lawyer as she rightfully got paid for a job well and honorably done. The real losers? You as patients are the losers, both from a monetary aspect, since in the end it is always the consumer who pays for lawsuits in direct or indirect ways, and from the perspective of the kind of medical care you are liable to receive. Let me explain.

Our legal system puts providers on high alert. We feel attacked on all sides. This state of anxiety inevitably leads to defensive medicine, which makes the doctor-patient relationship adversarial. Instead of the doctor making decisions on what is medically necessary, the doctor must first consider the legal consequences of every course of action.

Do you want a doctor who orders an extra $1,000 in tests so that she can protect herself from future lawsuits? Would you want the tests to prove/refute your doctor's theory, even though the chances are one in a million? Do you want a provider who puts the onus on you to make health care decisions for fear of making the *wrong* decision? Do you want a provider who sees you as a potential lawsuit? Or, do you want your provider to see you as a partner in your care?

As always, there are two sides to the coin. We must supply appropriate protections to health care providers so they know that, unless they genuinely commit malpractice, they can expect to be safeguarded from disgruntled and opportunistic patients. We also must protect patients from true malpractice so that you get the care you need.

Any meaningful discussion of bringing out-of-control medical malpractice to heel must include tort reform so that we can appropriately shield not only patients but also providers. Tort reform will reduce the high costs, financial and emotional, of malpractice (and other) lawsuits. Those who commit malpractice must be held to account, while those who do their best to deliver outstanding health care should enjoy a level of protection. Some state laws on this subject are reasonable, and some, not so much. We need to have federal oversight on tort reform to set a consistent standard for litigation. The savings will be enormous, as it's estimated that 2.4-10% of all health care spending is due to malpractice lawsuits and the defensive medicine that results from them![4] In the end, tort reform would benefit the most important person: YOU, the patient.

COMMON-SENSE SOLUTIONS:

- Malpractice lawsuits should only proceed if an independent body agrees that malpractice potentially occurred. If they deem it is possible, then the claim is credible. If the basis is frivolous, however, it is denied outright.
- The law should enforce a statute of limitations. Two years is more than a reasonable period to know if you have been injured and then to file a malpractice lawsuit.
- End-goals for malpractice lawsuits should be twofold: to make the injured person whole again (as much as money can make anyone "whole"), not rich; and to hold the provider accountable so that it does not happen again if they

---

4 Cauchi, Dick, et al. "Medical Malpractice Reform - Health Cost Containment." *Medical Malpractice Reform- Health Cost Containment, http://www.ncsl.org/research/health/medical-malpractice-reform-health-cost-brief.aspx (retrieved Dec 2019).*

"Of the people, by the people, for the people" - Abraham Lincoln

did commit malpractice. Reasonable limits on damages should be written into the law to help meet appropriate goals; again, not to make patients or lawyers rich off of the system.

- Lawyers' fees should be sensible. At no time should lawyers receive more than the individuals they represent.
- Different models of resolution should be encouraged rather than lawsuits.
- Whatever side loses should pay, not only for the legal fees but also for the lost wages and other reasonable expenses for the plaintiff (patient) OR the defendant (provider). This is only fair.
- If providers are found guilty, the medical board should be involved to determine a course of action to avoid further negligence. This is good policy; although, if the provider is found innocent, then all traces of the lawsuit should be stricken from their record. Similarly, if patients bring a reckless case forward, they should be held accountable, and it should be noted if they ever bring a lawsuit against another provider or any other citizen.

These are simple, common-sense solutions to help keep providers, patients, and lawyers liable for their actions and pay restitution to those who deserve it. Reform would also discourage frivolous lawsuits. By removing these external stressors, we can help remind providers of their original purpose in going into medicine—their "why"—which equates to better care and better access at a lower price from a friend, rather than a foe.

"Of the people, by the people, for the people" - Abraham Lincoln

AFTER ACTION REVIEW:

- Nobody wins when defensive medicine is practiced. It changes the nature of the doctor-patient relationship, so providers look at patients as potential adversaries, not partners. Only one side of this relationship is held accountable in a lawsuit—the provider. Research on your own, and understand tort reform as it relates to medical malpractice; then you can examine, and determine for yourself, what reasonable policies look like for all involved.

- Ask yourself, what is the purpose of malpractice litigation? Who benefits from the current system? I think you will find that it is not the patient, nor the provider, nor the system.

- How would you define our goals for health care in the USA?

- What are your personal health goals and what will you do TODAY to achieve them?

"Of the people, by the people, for the people" - Abraham Lincoln

NOTES:

NOTES:

CHAPTER 10

A PERFECT STORM

"Disease is the biggest money maker in our economy."
-John H. Tobe

TENET 1:
Optimal health frees people to secure, on their own terms, life, liberty, and the pursuit of happiness. Without health, our potential—both individually and societally—is blunted.

Feeling powerless lends little to favorable outcomes. Unfortunately, we incarcerate ourselves with powerlessness when we choose not to live purposefully with health in mind. This is a self-sustaining prison, fortified by a fee-for-service medical establishment that churns the perfect storm of our current health care system; it does not encourage health. Why? Because disease pays so well. More disease equals more fee-for-service charges, which means the entire health care system makes more money while costing the patient, you, more and more. Moreover, there are no incentives to prevent illness, so we think we are invincible until the prison's foundation begins to quake.

My patient Sam lived his life (without regard to his health) for seventy years. He enjoyed smoking, prolonged sun exposure, eating and drinking whatever he wanted. And for years, along with his other health care providers, I pressed upon him that he needed to start living a more healthful lifestyle.

"Doc, what is happening to me?" Sam asked. He sounded weak and slightly disgusted. "Look at my legs!"

"Well, you have a lot of pre-cancers and cancers on your legs from years in the sun. Also, after fifty years of smoking, the blood vessels in your legs have deteriorated to the point that they are not allowing anything to heal. That's the reason why the hair is no longer growing, the tissue is swollen, and nothing is recovering the way it should."

"I quit smoking five years ago!" His tone was skeptical, as if there was no part of him that could comprehend that the consequent power of fifty years spent smoking would still be at the root of his problems; after all, this was a long stretch of good behavior. That had to be enough.

"The damage is done," I said. "And while it is beneficial to stop smoking, I can't turn back the clock. I can't reverse the harm."

"So, what does this mean? Will I need to see you once or twice a month for the rest of my life? These cancers are coming faster than you can remove them. And nothing is healing!"

"Yes, you are growing skin cancers all over your body, and while we can't halt the progression, I can slow it down."

In an angry, disbelieving tone, Sam shot back, "But I don't want to live in your office!"

This is a familiar story for many patients, and I don't want that for you. There are options: you can either live a long, healthful life, determined and disciplined, or you can die slowly (and in miserable fashion). Sam did stop smoking five years ago. It was the only modification that he was willing to make. After years of abuse, his body would not bounce back any longer. This harm was irreparable. The effects translate to a rather unpleasant journey at the end of life as our bodies are no longer able to fight the onslaught of disease successfully.

No horror film is as scary, no words can describe to you, and no story can adequately relate how brutal the end-of-life health concerns are for those who have not consistently taken care of themselves throughout their lives. The momentum of health or disease that we create throughout life usually results in either a rather quick and dignified end for the healthy minority, or a continuous catastrophic collision with pain and suffering for the unhealthy majority. As any doctor will tell you, those who have taken care of themselves throughout life usually have a relatively comfortable last chapter compared to those who have abused their bodies. Why people refuse to take care of themselves usually stems from undiagnosed psychiatric disease, unhealthy emotional relationships with food, or mindsets that tell them that there are no consequences for actions, laziness, entitlement.

"Sam, that doesn't unmake the problem. Smoking has done irreversible damage to your blood vessels. If your circulation can't function properly, then the needed nutrients and oxygen are never delivered to your legs, and it can't carry away the waste that your body produces," I explained carefully and honestly. In essence, his legs were starving and suffocating while drowning in waste. "The edema in your legs is visible from across the room, and it is only nine in the morning. Your legs don't have good blood supply."

"If they will not heal, let's just let the cancers stay down there? Why should we even treat them?" Sam scoffed. "They don't bother me."

People have a fantastic tendency to put off the inevitable because they think that they are going to be the exception to the rule. They believe that relatively predictable and well-documented consequences will not arise for them. It is the type of thinking that says even though 40-50% of Americans will get divorced, you are convinced you never will.[5] You are going to be the unicorn, right? According to Sam's line of thinking, the unicorn part of the story is that he is going to be the magical exception, that everything is going to get better despite seven decades of deliberate action to the contrary.

Still, this story always ends the same for all with such delusions of invincibility: a horrible death that I would not wish upon history's worst villains. In the end, the patterns that bring patients to this point are the same patterns they revert to when they leave my office. They don't want to be proactive. They want to let sleeping dogs lie because no news is good news. We have all heard this defense, though, because there's always someone who smoked and drank and lived to be 101 years old. I have also heard that people often win the lottery; however, basing my retirement strategy on that statistical anomaly would be as smart as investing in tobacco futures as a doctor.

---

5 *American Psychological Association*, American Psychological Association, https://www.apa.org/topics/divorce

"Of the people, by the people, for the people" - Abraham Lincoln

Sam's thinking was flawed. I shook my head. "Right now, these are small squamous cell cancers, and if we do not treat them, they will produce wounds and nasty infections that are far worse than what you have now. They can spread internally. They eat you from the inside out, which will cause other, unattractive problems such as disability, disfigurement, and death. Likewise, we have already removed five melanoma skin cancers from your body over the last three years—and had we not treated them, they would have likely killed you by now." At this point I feel guilty as if these cancers were my doing. I feel guilty that no matter what we do to treat them, chronic wounds develop. Sam is starting to feel powerless, out of control, and angry. Much like me crouching down to the ground, gripping my weapon, and freaking out when the helicopter dropped me off at Camp Fallujah, Sam feels like he has no good direction to go in, can't see clearly through the fog of his medical reality, and does not know who is capable of hearing his concerns enough to change his destiny. He is lost, and I have absolutely no idea how to give him directions to a good destination.

"I agree with you, though," I admitted. "While there are treatment options for these cancers, we tried all of them over the last couple of years, and they produce chronic wounds that take months if not years to heal; these chronic wounds will be a cakewalk in the park compared to letting the cancers grow out of control. I do highly recommend we treat them. If you would like a second opinion, then I am happy to arrange one for you."

"Something has to be done," said Sam. "I refuse to live this way."

"Of the people, by the people, for the people" - Abraham Lincoln

For those with histories like Sam, the patient's indignation and obstinance are predictable. These are the predominant emotions displayed by patients in these situations because they can't assume the blame for how their lives have turned out. They cannot conceive that it's their fault.

Resentfulness will manifest, depending on where each person lives emotionally, in one of three ways. First, those who are prone to anger will turn on their health care provider; since their understanding of medicine is limited, they don't see why there isn't a magic potion to fix the natural outcome of an entire lifetime of neglect and abuse. Second, those with melancholy dispositions will feel distressed, lumping it together with their other misfortunes, and calling it "evidence" that the world is out to get them. And lastly, those who have the emotional intelligence to understand their part in their health care will assume the weight of their decisions, feeling grateful for whatever help they receive, and those people make plans of action. You do not have to be in medicine to know which personality type will cope with disease clinically, spiritually, and emotionally.

Sadly, a lifetime of poor choices has energy, and it is more than the measure of medicine to reverse and heal diseases formed over decades. Sam was barreling out of control on a trajectory he chose. He lit the match. He fueled it. He allowed the countdown to begin. And years later, there was little that anyone could do to regain control of a rocket that had already gone off.

Sam was now standing, trying to gain control of the situation. I was seated, leaning forward, and doing everything possible to communicate care and concern. The exam room was built for

"Of the people, by the people, for the people" - Abraham Lincoln

these types of encounters. The floors are eco-friendly wood laminate, the walls are a warm and inviting blue-gray, the artwork on the walls is breathtaking, the music calming, and everything is immaculate. It is a clinic designed to calm people down so that no matter what medically occurs in this hallowed office, every patient knows it was purpose built for them. But none of that mattered today. Today, the only thing that mattered was trying to turn fear into constructive action.

"I understand and am so sorry that all of this is happening. The vascular surgeon wanted to see if there was a way to increase circulation in your legs. At that time, there was really nothing else that they could do. Would you like me to see if anything has changed?"

My gaze fell. I felt bad for Sam. He was in a painful and challenging situation, and by that time, it did not matter who was at fault. Sam needed my help, but the therapeutic options were limited. Prevention was out. Maintenance of disease was the only path forward. Health was simply not possible anymore.

Sam snapped, "What the hell are they going to do?!" There was a quality of aggression in his voice—so strong that it stirred adrenaline into my blood. He was now invading my personal space and standing over me. I was still seated.

"I'm not sure, but they have expertise in an area that I do not. It's worth the visit." Sam didn't say anything, but his body language had a certain insight. With his anger, added to an equal dose of fear, the patient transformed himself and assumed the unpredictable stance of a wounded animal (not rational human). The pause extended, so I offered, "I could also send you

"Of the people, by the people, for the people" - Abraham Lincoln

to the University Dermatology Department in Denver to see if they have any other ideas—"

"What are they going to be able to do that is different? Or better?"

"A second opinion is often the best idea in difficult situations."

I often ask patients if they want a second opinion when the diagnosis or treatment plan is not relatively clear, though most patients reject the idea. They want to be told what to do; of course, they only want the advice that allows them to justify the current lifestyle that got them into this mess in the first place. If it's inconvenient, they will either ignore it, fight it, or vent to others that you are a horrible doctor who does not know what you are doing because you could not figure out a way to cure smoker's cough without quitting smoking. Seriously, 99 percent of people think they should be skinny, eat whatever they want, and never exercise. The other 1 percent are healthy individuals who don't need to see a doctor often. They live life on their terms because they appreciate that actions have consequences.

"I don't want to drive an hour to Denver," he retorted finally.

However, Sam just told me that he went up to Denver to pick up his wife at the airport; I knew it would not be a stretch for him to go again soon. Sam had a lifetime of poor patterns working to his detriment. All of them were mental. He did not want to address practical solutions because he was looking for something else—a wonderful way out—permission to live the way he wanted to live. The only problem is that he was no longer able to do so without serious intervention, because his body was about to fail...one organ system at a time.

"I could send you to another dermatologist in town, then."

"Of the people, by the people, for the people" - Abraham Lincoln

"I trust you, Doc! You have always taken good care of me. How many times have you saved my life now?"

He smiled, and I could feel his sincerity. But the sincerity was not in thanking me. Instead, his sincerity was pointed. He hoped that I would be able to present him with another course, a means to undo everything that was wrong with him.

There's a big difference.

I paused, then said, "I don't know, Sam. Are you willing to go back to the vascular surgeon or the wound clinic to see if they have anything to offer?"

"Last year, the wound clinic told me that you were doing everything they would do. Is there something that you're missing?"

"No, I think we need some help here—to keep you as healthy as possible. With everything going on with your legs, I think it's sensible to have other specialists weigh in and, at least, suggest some treatment possibilities."

There was a defining shift in our conversation, though it was subtle. When Sam asked how many times I had saved his life, the implication was that medicine's purpose was to rescue him. And now, it was medicine's responsibility (really, he saw it as my duty) to find a cure. Where is the patient's motivation to hold himself accountable? And why should he? No part of our medical system will challenge him, which places the burden on the provider, the nearest culpable subject, and when the patient inevitably gets sick, it will be someone else's job to remedy the situation. Medicine is the business of disease, after all.

Most patients in this situation are on Medicare because it takes years for the aftereffects of bad choices to set in. Then, it is society's responsibility to pay for their chronic care. Our system asks the same question over and over: "What pill can reverse a lifetime of poor health choices?" We want an easy, convenient, pain-free answer. It's the "get-rich-quick scheme" of medicine and it works as well in medicine as it does in real life. While people should not be forced to be healthy, society should not be forced to pay the bill for individuals who pursue an unhealthy standard of living.

But are we asking the wrong questions? We wonder, "What can medicine do for disease?" The answer we receive is disease and "death care" instead of what we truly need. Calling this "health care" is like calling global warming a "green solution to heating your home." We need better answers from medicine, so we need to ask better questions.

We need to know where to start.

"What can I do to be as healthy as I can be so that I need as little medicine as possible?" When we are healthy, we can be of service to ourselves and others. We can surpass our potential, and society's potential, by delivering complex solutions, and in the process, we will build individual legacies. Moreover, according to the Kaiser Family Foundation, the healthiest 50% of Americans only consume 3% of all health care costs. In other words, there are more than enough health care resources in this country if we would just do our part and make reasonable lifestyle choices.

I hope that this discussion will end this destructive process in which we concentrate on the wrong issues, neglecting to innovate for society's benefit. It is not what medicine can do for your

"Of the people, by the people, for the people" - Abraham Lincoln

disease—it's what you can do for yourself, your loved ones, and the world when you are healthy!

*****

Sam nodded at me. "I'll go to see the vascular gal, but I do not want to see another dermatologist."

"Understood. Do you have any more questions? Or should we start the procedure?" I asked gently.

"Doc, what choice do I have?"

It was rhetorical, a terse attempt to comprehend the truth and accept it: we were out of alternatives and we needed to proceed in treating one of his many cancers. The saddest piece is that he once had the power to control this cancer, but he squandered that. He chose the wrong path years ago, and continued, despite consistent warning signs. Finally, he arrived at the intersection of disease and death, not knowing in which direction he was headed.

Similarly, through decades of misguided public health policy and disingenuous legislation, the US has (not so proudly) come to the point of (successfully) delivering Universal Death Care in the Age of Entitlement.

WHERE DO WE STAND?

As Americans, we believe in our exceptionalism. We are the best at everything, right? Indeed, we should have the best health statistics in the world. Even among the wealthiest countries, we do not have the best longevity. In fact, for almost every single measure possible the US is worse than any other "similar" country like France, Canada, the UK, Switzerland, Norway, Japan, Spain, and Germany. The US has the highest percentage of GDP being spent on health care by a long shot, and we spend more per person on health care by a long shot, yet we have the same utilization rates of health care services as these other "similar" countries. We spend more on pharmaceuticals per capita and as a whole by a long shot, and we spend at least triple on health care administration costs as these other countries due to insurance company profits. So, if we are outliers on all of the above, we must have the best health outcomes compared to these "similar" countries, right? Wrong. For many measures, we are either the worst, or close to the worst for many health outcomes. Even when you account for the health of minorities and immigrants, America still has higher mortality, injury, and illness rates than the other "similar" nations. In other words, our system costs the most by a huge margin and has worse outcomes. Doesn't seem right.

Let's look at some of the markers of health while comparing the US to seventeen similar countries—our economic "peers"[6]: Americans die sooner. Americans have the highest infant mortality rates. We also rank poorly on most other infant health measures. We have a high homicide rate. Americans have higher rates of death from alcohol and drugs. We are the fattest country, with the highest number of patients with diabetes. We are

6 National Research Council (US); Institute of Medicine (US); Woolf SH, Aron L, editors.

Washington (DC): National Academies Press (US); 2013. "U.S. Health in International Perspective: Shorter Lives, Poorer Health."

"Of the people, by the people, for the people" - Abraham Lincoln

second for heart disease and death from heart-related causes. We lead in chronic lung disease and we also have a larger disabled population. It turns out that we are the best at producing an epic amount of disease and cost with worse outcomes.

For a country with more resources than any other, we have not done an excellent job of converting these resources into increased health for all Americans. Somehow, we have created a regurgitating situation in which we are among the unhealthiest. Bled dry by the system intended to help us, the only way to combat this crisis is for individuals to assume responsibility, prevent illness, and participate in their health care decisions personally, locally and nationally. Then, the government needs to step in and help the system support the health of all citizens. But first it starts with the citizens, as we are a country of the people.

Tenet 2:
Increasing the health of individuals will lead to a healthier, whole society.

As a child, my parents taught me many lessons. Some of them were by watching them be human, making their own mistakes, and some of them were helping me learn lessons as I messed up, all on my own. Sometimes the lessons were preemptive, as they foreshadowed my behavior and told me what would happen if I did X, Y, Z. Other lessons were in the form of punishment for making the wrong choices. And, sometimes, my parents did not have to teach me anything because it was blatantly obvious that the ramifications would be worse. Regardless, they held me accountable for my actions because they had my best interests at heart.

"Of the people, by the people, for the people" - Abraham Lincoln

We must regard public health policy in the same practical yet understanding way. There are times when people need to learn lessons themselves, times when people need to be warned about the consequences of their actions, and times when life will impose realities upon the participant. Unfortunately, the last of the learning strategies happens too late because of intractable disease. It's too late for the individual to change, to reclaim his or her health—too much damage has been done. There's not much to do as there is no "kill switch" for the ticking time bomb that has been in play for decades.

Again, by the time disease manifests, people are usually older, on Medicare, and it is the government's responsibility to carry the burden. First, public health policies must enable individuals to learn about their part in their health care, actively and passively, while teaching and motivating them to enhance their health. Individuals need to feel rewarded when they are eating nutritiously and exercising; conversely, they must also grasp the real-world consequences from an unhealthful lifestyle—before they even start to suffer and fight against it. They must understand the implications because poor choices must not just be felt, they must reverberate in the conscious mind. They have to be painful NOW; healthful decisions have to be rewarded NOW, or the time between deed and reward or penalty is just too far off to promote continually positive behaviors.

Let's take a look at a ridiculous hypothetical option of reward and penalty now or later (which is similar to Mischel's "Marshmallow Test"). If I were to poll a hundred 18-year-olds, which life path would they select from these two:

1) Rob a bank, enjoy life, filthy rich and in ridiculous luxury for the next forty-seven years. But then you'll get caught. You'll go to prison to pay for your crimes at 65 years old, forfeit your belongings, pay restitution, and you might not make it out alive. When you are old and free, you will have no hope of security or comfort.

2) Work hard, save your money, and put what you can into retirement funds. Be responsible for your entire life. At 65 years old, you will be financially independent, debt-free, and able to do almost anything you desire until your death.

How many 18-year-olds would pick Option 1? How many would go for Option 2? And there you have it. In a real sense, the majority of Americans choose present over future every day of their lives. Only about 10 percent of us consciously choose Option 2 every day (as it is a daily choice), which is why the system is failing. It can't handle the weight of self-indulgence, complacency, in addition to the lack of rewards and penalties. We need to change EVERYTHING from the inside out and lead the 90 percent toward Option 2. Imagine the world we would have. We could tap the potential of this great country if we all weren't so selfish and naively entitled, and took care of our future selves, now. Consider the following:

- In the US, the healthiest 50% of us will only consume 3% of total health care costs![7]

---

7 Sawyer, Bradley, and Gary Claxton KFF. "How Do Health Expenditures Vary across the Population?" *Peterson-Kaiser Health System Tracker*, https://www.healthsystemtracker.org/chart-collection/health-expenditures-vary-across-population/#item-discussion-of-health-spending-often-focus-on-averages-but-a-small-share-of-the-population-incurs-most-of-the-cost_2016.

"Of the people, by the people, for the people" - Abraham Lincoln

- 50-85% of all health care dollars are spent on diseases that are easily preventable—if people choose to live in a health-conscious manner (i.e., obesity, hypertension, diabetes, and high cholesterol levels).[8]
- In 2008, obesity alone cost $147 billion in medical costs and between $3.38 and $6.68 billion in absenteeism costs![9] That is the price of a single, chronic disease—and it's one that could largely be avoided. In 2015, about 40% of adults in the US were obese, while over 70% are overweight or obese![10] And we all know that the numbers of overweight and obese Americans increase every year. Staggering.
- Smoking-related costs total $300 billion per year![11]
- Diabetes-related costs totaled $245 billion in 2012.[12]
- To show that all the above diseases mostly present themselves with age, people over 55 years old account for over 50% of all health care spending, even though they represent only about 29% of the population.[13]

---

8 David M Cordani, "Infographic: From Sick Care to Health Care," Report Prepared for by Cigna, https://www.cigna.com/about-us/healthcare-leadership/from-sick-care-to-health-care-infographic (accessed July 21, 2019).

9 Cdc.gov. (2019). *Adult Obesity Causes & Consequences | Overweight & Obesity | CDC.* [online] Available at: https://www.cdc.gov/obesity/adult/causes.html [Accessed 20 Dec. 2019].

10 "FastStats." *Overweight Prevalence,* www.cdc.gov/nchs/fastats/obesity-overweight.htm. Accessed 20 Dec. 2019.

11 "Economic Trends in Tobacco." *Centers for Disease Control and Prevention,* 5 Dec. 2019, www.cdc.gov/tobacco/data_statistics/fact_sheets/economics/econ_facts/index.htm.

12 "Economic Costs of Diabetes in the U.S. in 2012." *PubMed Central (PMC),* 1 Apr. 2013, www.ncbi.nlm.nih.gov/pmc/articles/PMC3609540.

13 "How Do Health Expenditures Vary across the Population?" *Peterson-Kaiser Health System Tracker,* 21 Aug. 2019, www.healthsystemtracker.org/chart-collection/health-expenditures-vary-across-population/#item-discussion-of-health-spending-often-focus-on-averages-but-a-small-share-of-the-population-incurs-most-of-the-cost_2016.

"Of the people, by the people, for the people" - Abraham Lincoln

The numbers of people with these diseases are increasing every year because we, as a people, are growing more and more unhealthy. It is not hard to see that our poor health decisions are bankrupting our "health care" system. If we are not careful, we will be right there, along with Sam, living a predictable nightmare.

While Americans should have the right to be as healthy or unhealthy as they desire—that is, the total freedom to dictate their futures—we know that it comes with an array of consequences. Our car insurance rates go up if we drive carelessly, so should our insurance rates respond to those who are careless with their health when they are young and when they are old. Under our current system, the majority (over 70%) go into adulthood unaware of what it means to be healthy for an entire lifetime, and when it does come to their attention, the disease already has momentum (and they must entrust their lives to Medicare). This is not sustainable. Medicare's Board of Trustees has predicted that Medicare will run out of money by 2026! Along with other common-sense measures, we must find ways to reverse society's attitude toward health or make those who are unhealthy pay their fair share now for the future costs they will incur. We will fix it, or we will watch our medical system collapse.

COMMON-SENSE SOLUTIONS:

- We must provide abundant, universal, and free education, starting in elementary school and continuing throughout life, on how to be healthy. This education must be complete, accurate, easily digested, readily available to all, and free from commercial bias.

"Of the people, by the people, for the people" - Abraham Lincoln

- If we are not responsible consumers, then we must pay more now to help cover anticipated increased health care costs in the future.

AFTER ACTION REVIEW:

- Ask yourself to take an honest survey of your health. Are you doing the things that are necessary for you to live un-encumbered by preventable diseases? Does your lifestyle encourage disease? Which ones? Take note of what you have done well and not so well for your health this past week. Be specific.Write down a plan for what you will do better for your health this next week. Make a tangible plan, take it upon yourself to do the research, ask for help if you need to, and do it! One step at a time will complete a very worthwhile journey.

"Of the people, by the people, for the people" - Abraham Lincoln

NOTES:

NOTES:

CHAPTER 11

THERE IS NO ENEMY HERE

"For the strength of the pack is the wolf, and the strength of the wolf is the pack."
-Rudyard Kipling, *The Jungle Book*

QUESTION:
What do you consider the most consumed drugs on the planet?

Answers:
A) Pain medications as a class (aspirin, ibuprofen, prescription and illegal narcotics)
B) Mind-altering substances as a class (alcohol, nicotine, caffeine)
C) Blood pressure medications as a class
D) Weight-loss drugs and supplements (sports drinks, protein powders, prescriptions)
E) Other

Please circle your choice before continuing…the truth will be revealed later.

Tenet 3:

While an individual should not be required to make a speci-fied set of healthful choices, each person should take responsi-bility for the sum of those choices; at the same time, the group should not be penalized for an individual's decision (such as rationing of care and/or resources).

Remember the last time you walked into a dining room and knew, immediately, that you were the main course? You may have dreaded it, or they may have sprung it on you, but you felt as though you'd been carved up and roasted along with dinner. Unfortunately, this is an all too familiar scenario in medicine.

For me, it was the surprise of walking into a surgical room, a medical student by my side, when a familiar and unnecessarily aggressive scene began. Something else was going on. It was pal-pable in the air. Understanding the importance of first impression and presentation as we entered the room, I introduced myself and Amy with a smile and then finished with a sincere handshake.

The room chilled. The mother already had her arms crossed.

She's in charge, I noticed. Satisfying her demands would be a priority; she was already angry. While the father was disinter-ested, he showed dominance by assuming the awkward posture of someone who has watched too many amateur flexing videos on YouTube. He hardly acknowledged us. He briefly glanced up from his phone, legs spread out and posture hunched, and it was immediately apparent that we all were in for an unpleasant ride. The patient, the son, was acting like a typical teenager in this situ-ation—distant and uncertain about what was about to happen to him.

"Hi, my name is Dr. Anderson," I greeted them warmly. "But most people call me Reagan. This is Amy, and she is a third-year medical student." Even if you weren't looking in my direction, you'd still hear the smile in my voice.

The family also introduced themselves, each revealing their emotional state. There was silence. The father, who was sprawled out and lounging in a chair, gave a quick, unintentional hand-shake, only to refocus on his phone. He couldn't care less about what was happening.

"Are there any questions about what we are doing or why we are doing it?" As this was our pre-surgical meeting, the parents had supposedly watched our videos on the procedure, read and signed the consent, and agreed to the verbal consent. Instead of acknowledging the question or the one who was asking, the room quietly turned away from me. An angry mother. A distant father. And a passive-aggressive, surly teenager.

At that point, I decided to re-explain the diagnosis from the pathologist's report with the recommendation to remove this atypical mole. There was another atypical mole near the one we were excising, and though we biopsied that site, there was no need to remove it. The mother asked me how large the excision would be, so I proceeded to prep the area with alcohol and drew the borders. After we took a picture of it, the family looked at a picture of the patient's back while I started explaining the surgery.

"You need to remove both moles today," the mother inter-rupted. "They are *close enough.*"

I tried to show her that while the moles might be close, about three inches apart, they were not directionally located for a healthy outcome. That would make a one-and-a-half-inch scar closer to eight inches. There was no medical justification to do so, given the diagnosis and the recommendations of the pathology report.

The mother was righteous and indignant, waving her hand at me and proceeding as though I was put on this earth for her amusement. Amy and I left the room so that my staff could prep the area for surgery.

In the hallway, Amy took a deep breath to say, "That was unbelievable. The mother needs everyone to know she is Momma Bear."

After over 35,000 surgeries, the task of removing an atypical mole is relatively straightforward. Dealing with the emotional end is not. You are concerned, not with the patient's cancer, but with their baggage—placating their egos, being more interested in their health than they are, and putting up with these needlessly negative and aggressive situations. Does rudeness to another human being yield better results when you order food at a restaurant? Or when a police officer pulls you over? Yet, if you ask anyone in health care about their day, they will likely recall a half-dozen encounters from that day alone.

Providers "Embrace the Suck" because a health care professional's prime directive is to help people. We are there to help, so there is little we can do to stand up for ourselves when facing disgruntled patients. Our mission has nothing to do with that. Health care professionals are, sadly, punching bags in society. We provide hostile bullies a place to hunt. We are not protected legally. We can't respond to negative reviews posted online be-

"Of the people, by the people, for the people" - Abraham Lincoln

cause that would violate HIPAA. We can't unionize to protect ourselves or advocate for our patients because that would give us too much power. We can be sued for literally anything, and while most judges dismiss these lawsuits without merit, the ensuing damages and defensive medicine are costly for everyone involved. Our only course of action is to do our best and try to avoid verbal abuse as often as possible.

The mother's actions did not speak to her decision-making skills. She made her son into a scapegoat—a way for her need to take out her stress. If the mother had genuine concern for her son, then she would have behaved differently. The father was present; however, it also seemed like he was there under duress and made it his job to make everyone as miserable as he was. There were three patients in that room: one surgical and two psychiatric. The mother was anxious about satisfying her emotional need for attention while the father's primary goal was to intimidate. The son just wanted it to be over with as soon as possible.

Remember the last time someone aggressively confronted you? Put yourself there now. Go ahead. Put the book down and spend thirty seconds reliving that experience so you can feel the situation as a recent event.

Is your blood pressure elevated? Are your hands steady? Is your thinking clear? Are you in the optimal state to do your job—whatever it might be? If the answer is no, then why would people deliberately try to put their doctor in that state before a procedure or an office visit?

Amy and I went to talk with another patient, but before we could, we had to let the past situation go. Bringing negativity into the next room would only keep us from being present and available, which is why the knock on the next door is programmed into my subconscious as a reset button. This sound means my soul has anywhere from thirty seconds to a couple of minutes to get over situations like what just happened. Then I am never going to bring it up again. If I held on to these meetings to rehash them later, nonsense would overload my memory; I'd become the sullen, peevish father—not the helper I am meant to be. And, if I ever become that emotionally stunted or as purposely selfish, then I need to remove myself from this career and retire to an island where I can work on critical self-development.

Knock, knock.

After seeing another patient, Amy and I took a deep breath, reframing our attitudes to a surgically conducive state, and walked back into the cold surgical room (after hitting the reset button). With smiles and interest, we said hello to everyone again and asked if they were ready to start the procedure. They didn't even grunt.

During these procedures, I always talk to my patients, educating them, answering questions, and telling stories or jokes... anything to put them at ease. It's a stressful operation for many patients, so talking helps the time pass quickly, and usually it has a calming effect. If the surgical team does not engage the patient during a procedure, then silence takes over the patient—awake, and without any sedation—who becomes nervous. The patient allows his mind to wander, and he wonders if the procedure is going so poorly that we need to concentrate all our efforts on the problem at hand.

"Of the people, by the people, for the people" - Abraham Lincoln

"Please, do not let the area get wet with water or sweat, for two days," I recited. "The area on top of your son's shoulder needs time to get watertight—before any moisture tries to infect the wound."

The mother balked at this. "What?! He can't shower for two days?"

"No, he can shower," I offered carefully. "Just shower from the waist down so that we can keep this area dry for a couple of days."

"Ridiculous. He's not doing that," she said.

"Please, do not do *any* exercises or activities that will put direct pull or pressure on the wound for six weeks, so it has a chance to heal before being bothered or stretched."

While these instructions were already explained to them multiple times and in various formats leading up to the surgical appointment, this seemed like new information.

"What about basketball?" the father asked without glancing up.

And I shook my head. "Basketball for the next six weeks is not a good idea. If we put too much stress on a fresh surgical wound, the outcome will not be good. The scar will spread, or it could rip open. It might bleed or get infected. It can cause other problems as well."

"He plays basketball, and he's not taking six weeks off." The father's tone was impersonal and icy.

The mother joined him, "That's not reasonable for something so small! He will take two days off. But that is it!"

"I understand your concerns. My job is to inform you what

I think will be the best practice for the best outcome, based on experience. Does anyone have any questions about the suggestions? You will also get a printed handout. There are videos on our website, www.coderm.com, that will explain post-surgical care."

"You seriously want him to stop playing basketball for six weeks?" the father continued to argue.

"Yes, sir," I said. "That is my recommendation."

*****

Tenet 4:

Health care must be just. We need reasonable legal and administrative protections for our providers. We need to advocate for doctors so that they are supported in practicing essential medicine and not the defensive medicine that is also potentially invasive (and costly).

Health care providers should not be held responsible for how quickly the human body can heal, nor should they be blamed for the factors controlled by the patient, which are seldom followed. They should not be held accountable when the patient does not follow simple directions. And yet, the way things are now, the only party held accountable in the medical system is the provider. This one-sided scheme has stretched into every corner of medical care. Each year, this flawed thinking leads to higher costs, poor results, and unbelievable frustration.

For instance, insurance carriers will punish providers if their patients do not achieve better control of their blood pressure, and though this seems sensible at first, a practical approach shows that the doctor's role is constrained:

1)   Usually, patients must commit to losing excess weight through appropriate diet and exercise.

2)   Patients need to watch what they eat, curbing their salt intake and avoiding fried or processed foods that increase inflammation in the body. They also need to consume certain foods, like fruits and vegetables, to ensure absorption of nutrients.

3)   Patients need to consistently take their medications.

4)   Patients must actively manage their stress.

5)   Patients need to get enough sleep.

6)   Patients need to return to the clinic for further testing and follow-up.

A provider's insight can't control anything on this list, but if the patient does not achieve a specified drop in blood pressure, the provider is penalized. We are not independent. We are all in this together. It's as ridiculous as holding one driver accountable for the speed of the cars surrounding him. Still, the government, endeavoring to save money, puts the onus of achieving lower blood pressure on the provider, who has little control over the outcome. A reasonable form of accountability for the provider would address medication, education on the contributing factors for hypertension, orders for appropriate blood work (to make sure that nothing else is going on that needs attention), and follow-up with the patient.

However, when the government makes providers liable for the patient's actions, without doing the same for the patient, it is an abuse of power, at worst, and the proof of the system's ineptitude, at best.

Having been a doctor for seventeen years, let me tell you what the above surgical patient will do:

1) He'll allow unclean water to wash over the wound within a couple of hours.

2) He will start playing basketball within a day or two.

3) The wound will not heal well, which will develop a large scar that will someday need to be revised when he has gained some wisdom (and when he's outside his parents' influence).

4) The parents will blame his provider for an adverse outcome, demand a meeting with me to say that I did an awful job, and publish a negative review online. Maybe, there will be more severe consequences for me. One thing I have learned in medicine is that the guiltier someone is, the more they will try to force somebody else to pay for it.

"Okay. We're all done here. Amy is going to get you bandaged and give you directions for care. Any questions?" I paused for a reply, and when there was none, I said goodbye, thanked my assistant for her help and left the room. We then prepared to see our next patient. Both Amy and I wondered what emotional smörgåsbord was waiting behind the next *knock, knock.*

*****

Tenet 5:
Every piece of the health care system must be held to account, not just the provider.

"Of the people, by the people, for the people" - Abraham Lincoln

Checks and balances are necessary within the health care system. Medical malpractice needs rational reforms to accomplish this goal, and while patients should have the right to file suit, the checks and balances should apply to the rest of the system. Why was this scene with my patient's family so contentious? Why did his parents refuse to read the consent, watch the videos on how to prepare for the surgery, or listen to my aftercare instructions? What keeps patients from participating in their side of their health care? Before you pass on to the next chapter, I want to ask, when was the last time you had a procedure? Did you read the consent form? Did you read the package insert for that new prescription? And when did you review and understand your insurance contract?

The point is that the more you, the reader, abdicate your responsibility to actively participate in your health care, the more control the medical system will hold over you. In denying your attention to these issues, you set yourself up for failure—be it medical, emotional, or financial.

To further illustrate this point, we should shift to the topic of drugs. American citizens consume more prescription medications than anyone else on the planet, per capita. We pay more for our prescriptions, and we also have some of the worst health outcomes of any country on Earth. It all stems from lack of culpability from everyone in the system, starting with you and carrying on to the administrators of medical schools, insurance companies, pharmaceutical companies, disingenuous lobbyists, government rules and regulations. A lack of engagement by the populace is what has allowed an entire system to fracture. No

"Of the people, by the people, for the people" - Abraham Lincoln

one wants to pay attention. It is entitlement at its worst. We expect to be taken care of without doing what we need to do, learn what we need to learn, vote what is best for the country. When a democracy no longer cares about the direction its country is headed in, then that leaves a power vacuum that corporations and government will use to their advantage.

Tenet 6:
One should have abundant access to resources that promote wholesome choices.

First, let's examine the concepts of drugs. It's more than just prescriptions. Drugs can be anything that induces a physiological, including psychological, change in the body when ingested or when they come in contact with the body. As such, the answer to the question of "What is the most consumed drug on the planet" is E) Other. Specifically, food is the most commonly consumed drug, as food induces physiological and psychological change. We need to address the drug industry, demanding how the populace can conduct checks and balances.

My practice requests prior authorizations (permission from an insurance company to do something) for procedures, referrals, and medications. By definition, this is the standard of care that I have been learning about and figuring out for almost two decades. That's the whole purpose of medical school, residency, continuing medical education, and the provider's practical experience. That's our job—to determine the best route, and we are more than held accountable when we get it wrong. Of course, the "best route" is for us to prevent disease in the first place, not just write a script to mask the symptoms. Regardless, when we prescribe a treatment course we somehow get rejected over and over, all day long by a "system" that is designed to save money, not lives.

Not long ago, I removed cancer from a woman's upper lip, then reconstructed her lip after we obtained clear margins. Since the cancer was bigger than I had anticipated, the reconstruction was more significant, but when I wrote a script for pain medication (a generic) for post-surgical pain, her insurance denied my request. Her plan denied *ALL* pain medications. We filled out the paperwork for a prior authorization for a pain medication, which was urgently needed, but the delayed response from the insurance would be at least two days. It would be a rejection. After many back-and-forth communications with the insurance company, the five-day supply for pain relief was refused. She ended up paying around $50 to get the Vicodin herself, and while we averted the worst situation, we did not solve the problem. Why do insurance companies abuse their ability to deny medications? Because they can. And the longer they hold on to their money, the more they make in interest. Who will stop them? This is the shared experience for health care providers around the country, so where are the lawsuits taking on the insurance companies? I'm sure they exist, though I can't remember the last time I heard about one. The sad truth is that insurance companies can do whatever they want, whenever they want—with little practical oversight or accountability, other than to make money.

There was another patient whose scalp was being eaten away by a fungal infection. He just needed a medication called Terbinafine that had been generic for years. I ordered the drug, his insurance company turned me down; instead, they would permit me to write a script for Ketoconazole (it can cause acute liver damage/failure and eventually, the FDA had to tell the industry to use it as a last resort). The better medication was Terbinafine, $4 a script, in cash, at the local pharmacy. I spent an hour trying to get a prior authorization because it was a matter of principle—who were they to deny this? They hung up on me three times, each time saying we were cut off. They never approved it. The patient ended up paying the $4.

On other occasions, I have been laughed at when I ordered a CT scan for a patient who may or may not have had brain tissue poking out of an opening in his skull. I needed to make sure that was not the case, in this particular location, and verify that it was a cyst before performing a surgery to remove the mass. It was denied. This has to stop.

Is the requirement for doctors to get prior authorizations worth it? Do they increase the quality of care and save everyone money? What good is a medical degree when a drone, hired by the insurance company, has the power to refuse a medical necessity? And that delay has consequences! Is that sound logic? Or is this just another method by which insurance companies increase their profits by denying care? Their industry claims that prior authorizations benefit patients, as a safety net, which will make sure that the physicians are practicing appropriate medicine. Why, then, do they often go against the standard of care? Why would these companies contradict what the medical community agrees is fitting, or common practice? It doesn't matter if they've chosen a reason. What is right, recommended, and what is customary has more to do with your insurance, what limits they have placed on treatments and tests, and how much you pay than it does with anything else. More than 90% of physicians surveyed by the American Medical Association (AMA) say that prior authorizations will affect patient care negatively. If this is not the rationing of care, then I don't know what is. This has to stop.

A *Health Affairs* study in 2009 sought to determine how much providers interacting with insurance companies was costing providers. They found that on average, it costs $68,274 per physician per year to cut through the red tape of insurance companies so that patients can get the care they need and physicians can get paid for their services. Each year in the USA, this totals between $23 and $31 billion that providers spend to fight with insurance companies in order to advocate for their patients to get the tests, procedures, and therapies they need in order to get better! Not a penny should need to be spent advocating for the patient to get standard-of-care medicine, let alone $23-31 billion. Like all things in business, the rise in price is passed down directly to the consumer, which means that not only are these companies doing everything possible to decrease the medicine you are allowed to consume, but you are also paying them to deny your care. The only way this will change is if we start educating ourselves, understanding how the consequences of the system's flaws, things like prior authorizations, have hurt you or your loved ones.

Another common issue is that industry artificially raises its prices. We all remember the EpiPen scandal of 2017. The company boosted the price of an EpiPen by over 500%, then hired a ton of lobbyists to ensure its products made it into the schools in many states. Because of its use in emergency medicine, this life-saving medication was taken away and placed out of reach of those who needed it most. Like the current price-gouging on insulin, greed fueled this scandal, and ultimately, the company paid a hefty price (after Congress got involved). But EpiPen is not exceptional; it's just a case, singled out and well-publicized. In truth, the pharmaceutical companies have been playing these games for years. The mean cost of Doxycycline (a generic anti-biotic that has been available for decades) "increased from $7.16 in 2011 to $139.89 in 2013, a 1,854% increase," and there were NO market forces found to explain this price increase.[14] It did not come to Congress' attention, the press decided it was not worth noting, and since the media decides what is on the po-litical agenda, nothing happened. According to the research di-vision of GoodRx, a month's supply of Xarelto (the third most common prescription anticoagulant) has gone up 54% over the past six years; Humira (for arthritis and psoriasis) cost $2,914/month in 2014, now it's $5,174/month—a 78% increase. These grave examples are too numerous to list. It has to stop.

Pharmaceutical companies consider increasing the costs of their drugs less than 10% a year an "acceptable" increase. Where is the logic or empathy in that? If inflation is 1-2%, why is a 9.9% increase a year considered "acceptable"? From the perspec-tive of the pharmaceutical company, however, there are no limits

---

14 "A 1,854% Price Hike." *Dermatology Times*, www.dermatologytimes.com/acne-treatment-and-compliance-resource-center/1854-price-hike. Accessed 29 Dec. 2019.

"Of the people, by the people, for the people" - Abraham Lincoln

placed on them other than what the market will bear. They have the perfect moneymaking machine because they provide a product that saves lives daily, and people will die if they don't hand over the money to use it. President Trump used to think that the government should negotiate medical prescription costs; he was looking to put in legislation to reverse part of the Medicare Modernization Act of 2003, which did not allow the government to negotiate drug prices. Now, President Trump does not think that the government should be allowed to do this—not even for Medicare, a government-run program. It boggles the mind to put a limitation on the government (not able to negotiate prices) that no private business could survive if they had the same restrictions. I thought President Trump was supposed to be a good businessman. The lack of appropriate laws to protect patients means that drug prices will significantly outpace inflation. We spend more on health care and on pharmaceuticals per capita in the USA than any other similar country. Yet we do not have the best health outcomes.

Further, a 2019 study from the Kellogg School of Management at Northwestern University found that Canadians pay 56% less than we do for the exact same prescriptions, because they negotiate prices! Perhaps it is time to limit the lobbyists' influence, force politicians to care more about the people than getting funding for their next election, educate those who make public policy that the ability to negotiate is good business, and pass some reasonable legislation so that pharmaceutical companies can still profit and innovate while not sacrificing patients' health. The only way this will change is if we stand up and demand to be heard at least as much as the corporations are.

The government also favors corporations when it comes to public health. It has not limited the industries contaminating our food and drinking water, which, in turn, causes disease; American laws are insufficient, and we are lax in our efforts to reverse the damage. The weed-killer RoundUp has lost its lawsuits. RoundUp has been banned in countries around the world and research shows that it is most likely a cancer-causing agent in humans; yet, the EPA refuses to ban its use until they can conduct further studies to determine its safety. Why is the EPA neglecting its purpose—to protect the public? Why does the FDA allow hundreds of toxic ingredients in our cosmetic products while other developed nations are banning them? This quotation is from the FDA website: "With the exception of color additives and a few prohibited ingredients, a cosmetic manufacturer may use almost any raw material as a cosmetic ingredient and market the product without an approval from FDA."[15] The EU bans 1,328 chemicals from cosmetics due to safety concerns. In the US? Eleven![16] These cause cancer and congenital disabilities. I thought we established the EPA and the FDA to protect Americans from consuming harmful products? Pick up an item from your bathroom closet, then go to the Environmental Working Group website, www.ewg.org, to see what the effects are of the

---

15 Center for Food Safety and Applied Nutrition. "Cosmetics Safety Q&A: Prohibited Ingredients." *U.S. Food and Drug Administration*, FDA, https://www.fda.gov/cosmetics/resources-consumers-cosmetics/cosmetics-safety-qa-prohibited-ingredients. Accessed 14 Dec. 2019.

16 "International Laws." *Safe Cosmetics*, http://www.safecosmetics.org/get-the-facts/regulations/international-laws. Accessed 12/14/2019.

"Of the people, by the people, for the people" - Abraham Lincoln

substances you've been slathering on your skin. You will be both amazed and horrified at what is allowed in this country. Perhaps it is time the FDA looked after our health instead of allowing corporations to sell snake oil, only to make more money. Our voices can effect change if we learn the system's flaws, vote at the ballot box and vote with our wallets. But first, we have to get educated. Then we have to care enough to make things better for the next generation.

In addition to cosmetics and pesticides, did you know that food is also made and marketed, regardless of the harmful health effects? The major food manufacturers hire teams of scientists to determine how to make foods addictive to ensure that you consume more. Unfortunately, the ingredients that make a food addictive are not nutritious. The opposite is true. Chemists spend their entire careers searching for ways to engineer foods that keep us from feeling full—they want us to keep consuming their product—and that is where their job ends. Sound is also important. If a snack "crunches," we will consume more. All of these ultra-processed foods are killing us, literally. A 2019 study found that if you consume more than four ultra-processed foods (cereals, breakfast bars, energy drinks, soda, crackers) in a day, your chances of dying (from all causes) go up 62%. For each additional serving, your risk will go up another 18%![17] Scary? Yes. How many ultra-processed foods did you consume today? The big food manufacturers are legal drug dealers who kill more people every year than illicit substances do. Yet, how are we

---

17 Rico-Campa et al., Association between the consumption of ultra-processed foods and all cause mortality: SUN prospective cohort study. BMJ 2019 May 29; 365.

holding those companies to account when they're poisoning us slowly and making a mint doing it?

Health care providers are and must continue to be responsible for their actions, and it must be equal to the other factors that affect one's health. Where is the accountability for insurance companies? How much responsibility should Big Pharma shoulder? Is it worth asking our politicians these questions, or is it just that everyone else has the money to hire the lobbyist who can sway the vote, and nobody can represent the needs of the average citizen because they no longer care, or even approach their own health care choices with a degree of concern? If the greatest American corporations can buy a democracy, then is it still a government for the people and by the people? Or is it oligarchy? What hope is there for substantive change? Or have we shut ourselves out?

Tenet 7:
Disease prevention must be the highest priority.

The health care industry does not want Americans to be healthy. They want us to be absolutely sick because sickness drives profits. This has to stop. Personal responsibility must be a priority, and corporate and government responsibility must rise to meet it. The only way this will happen though is for citizens to stand up and become involved. The system must be of the people, by the people, for the people, but for this to happen, we must show up. I am not advocating for socialism here, as the evils of socialism are just as perverse as capitalism when they are unchecked, unaccountable, and unsustainable. I am advocating

"Of the people, by the people, for the people" - Abraham Lincoln

for sound policy that is as sensitive to the individual's freedom as it is for checks and balances on unfettered greed.

Tenet 8:
Advancements in health care knowledge and delivery should be encouraged, regardless of profitability.

Tenet 9:
Health care needs to be affordable, accessible, and sustainable.

Tenet 10:
Common sense, not overly obtrusive strategy, needs to rule.

Tenet 11:
The system cannot tolerate fraud, waste, or the abuse of resources.

Medicine is necessary for life. We will all need medical care at some point. While there is room for capitalism within the medical system, we all need to keep watch individually, societally, and governmentally, without exploiting the patient when the patient does not have a way to combat abuse. We must fight for the patient's right to get medical care in an affordable and sustainable manner. You must stand up for your rights, too, which means being informed and caring enough to show up as well as having sound policies that are easy to understand. We must fight against only one side of the equation being held accountable. We must fight for protections for health care providers who are doing good work for patients who have other agendas. We must take action, or the other elements in the system will push for profits at the expense of everything else.

*****

Tenet 12:
Public health policy should encourage the entire population to take responsibility for their own health—blind to social influences while attentive to educational, regional, and cultural nuances.

Though I wasn't sure when the teenager and his parents would return to the clinic for a surgical site evaluation, I was dreading it. I did my best work in caring for his family. At the end of the day, how well the patient obeys directions will determine how well he heals. Instead of creating enemies with the provider, and instead of an industry trying to exploit people to satisfy their stockholders, instead of governmental policy being dictated by the highest bidder, maybe we should change the aim of our compass, recognize each other as the friends we are, and help each other achieve health. Perhaps, when we see that we could be allies, we will start to comprehend how we are connected. What is healthful for society is beneficial for the individual. What is nourishing for the individual is advantageous for the corporations since they consist of people. And what is healthful for the individual will also make the government capable of supporting its citizens. We are all in this together, and there is no enemy other than the enemy of greed, selfishness, entitlement and apathy—a combination that destroys anything in its path.

"Of the people, by the people, for the people" - Abraham Lincoln

Tenet 13:
We should not sacrifice our rights and freedoms to implement health care policy.

Tenet 14:
Health care is not a partisan issue, and as such, partisan power-plays have no role in the discussion.

Tenet 15:
Health care policy in the US needs to be constitutionally sound and supported by every branch of the government.

The strength of the US lies in our citizens, and the power of the citizens lies in our freedoms. We must be allowed to live healthy lives in order to experience the independence to pursue our dreams. It's time that the government got to work protecting our rights instead of creating laws that purely support industry. There is no price tag on freedom—some things are priceless—but right now, we, as citizens of this great country, are silent in the provider's office, silent when signing insurance contracts, silent at the pharmacy, and silent at the ballot box. There is no mystery here, just tragedy.

There is a toxic and unsustainable imbalance in the health care system caused by ill-considered, uninformed, and counterproductive government policies and partisan nonsense on the part of the government, greed and disingenuous influence on the part of the corporations, and confusion, entitlement, and apathy on the part of the patients; in addition, there is burnout and defensive medicine on the part of providers. All of the above

"Of the people, by the people, for the people" - Abraham Lincoln

are causing distrust of the government, contempt for the corporations, and harm to the patients. Nobody is winning.

COMMON-SENSE SOLUTIONS:

- Get involved, get educated, and let your voice be heard. Stop being helpless by design. It's that simple!

AFTER ACTION REVIEW:

- Write down how personally responsible you have been in your health care. Do you read the consent forms? Do you read through your insurance contracts? Do you understand what is happening to you and why? Are you voting for candidates who are taking this topic seriously...and are you holding them accountable for their campaign promises? Are you a responsible citizen?
- Write down what from the above bullet point needs to change, today, and how you will do so going forward.

"Of the people, by the people, for the people" - Abraham Lincoln

NOTES:

NOTES:

CHAPTER 12

PUTTING YOUR HEAD IN THE SAND ONLY MAKES IT HARDER TO BREATHE

"Unless we put medical freedom into the Constitution, the time will come when medicine will organize itself into an undercover dictatorship."
-Benjamin Rush

I took a plane to my first medical school interview, feeling incredibly awkward and wondering who in the world would see "doctor" potential in me. With oversized glasses and a face full of acne, I sat next to an attractive middle-aged woman, curious about my travel plans. When she learned where I was going and that I was applying to medical school, the conversation segued in a strange direction. She reached into her purse and pulled out a portfolio of pictures of her daughter, then extolled her beauty, her intelligence, her sense of humor. And she was available. By the end of the ride, I was not quite sure I was happy with the name of our first child, but I reasoned that there would be time to negotiate such trivial things.

During that first month of medical school, I walked into a coffee shop to study and noticed a table full of young women looking at me as if I were a piece of meat. While deciding on what cut they wanted, they kept peering over a newspaper, then looked down, and back up to me. Since I didn't know anyone in this small town, apart from the other medical students, this felt odd. I didn't yet know how often it would repeat itself.

Nervously, I sat down with my classmates and, at the risk of breaking the code of study silence, I wondered aloud if there was anything unusual in how the girls were looking at us as though they knew us. They laughed and slid the newspaper across the table to show me the spread: the newspaper published all the new medical school students' pictures, including mine. The locals who expected the students to arrive in town would begin selecting their "marks" soon—and they would pursue us with vigor.

At graduation, my grandfather approached me with an air of reverence and shook my hand, congratulating me, "Dr. Anderson. You are the first doctor in our family. How does it feel?"

Honestly, it felt just like the previous birthdays when he had asked me how it felt to be a year older—the same way as I felt five minutes ago. There was no divine light from above, shining on everything I did. There was no secret knowledge passed down via a sacrificial medical school education to the gods of health. I did not hear God whisper in my ear, telling me how to heal others. I didn't even get a decoder ring to translate medical jargon that was not yet really understood. I was the same: insecure, scared, in debt and a bit hungover from the previous night.

For my grandfathers, it meant the world. They placed more faith in doctors than in God, and when we had conversations about it over the years and I explained what doctors were and

"Of the people, by the people, for the people" - *Abraham Lincoln*

were not, they would not (or could not) understand my point of view. They never spoke to me or looked at me the same after graduation because, after all, I was a doctor.

I did not understand it seventeen years ago, but I do now. People need to have faith when they feel out of control. They find it in religion, in money, in science, and some find it in their doctors, but that is part of the human condition—we need to put our faith in something constant in order to navigate the uncertain world.

Many patients look at doctors as if we are chosen—each one of us motivated by a divine blessing, which is a superpower—and we have the backing of irrefutable science to guarantee concrete outcomes. Nothing could be further from reality. We are humans. We are doing our best with the knowledge and resources available. On the first day of medical school, they told us, "Medical school is like trying to take a drink through a fire hose. Fifty percent of what we are teaching you is completely wrong. The problem is that we don't know which fifty percent is incorrect." There is just too much information, with too much uncertainty with too many variables for us to really know what is accurate and should be swallowed and what is garbage and should be regurgitated. It's a hard truth. Just like millions of Americans, we are frequently winging it with our recommendations. Sure, there is a lot of research, hard work, and good intent behind everything we do. But, make no mistake—we are practicing. Even with lab results and fancy equipment and a perfect diagnosis, we can sometimes do nothing more than make an educated guess about that most complicated machine, the human mind, body, and spirit—the Trinity of Health that must be considered with every encounter, diagnosis, and treatment. The older the model of the machine and the more the machine has been abused, the more attention it needs.

"Hello, Sam. Good to see you."

"Wish I could say the same, Doc," Sam replied with a friendly but half-hearted smile.

"I know. I wish there weren't another cancer either, but hopefully, this will be easy to remove. Any questions about what we are going to do today or why we are doing it?"

"No, Doc. *I trust you.* This isn't my first rodeo, you know?"

We trust our doctors because we have a fundamental belief in their profession: they want us to be healthy. We mistakenly believe that all aspects of the system are working in tandem. We cannot see how incongruent that is.

Tenet 7:
Disease prevention is the highest priority.

At first, it's confidence-building when patients say that they trust you as their doctor, and still, at first, you take the compliment because you suppose that they are a good judge of your dedicated, dependable, and capable character. You might enjoy these types of encounters because it makes you feel like you are the Health Superhero, complete with an official title, fighting against your arch-nemesis, Disease. At first, it's impossible to tell what is behind such verbal expressions of trust, but there is a nasty underbelly to those comments in every profession; watch out for the implications attached to such statements!

"Of the people, by the people, for the people" - Abraham Lincoln

Back in the room with Sam, I paused, looking him in the eye and saying, "Well, let me clean the area where we took the biopsy, then I will ask you to confirm the location."

This is a "time out," where the provider finds the lesion's location, asks for confirmation from the patient, confirms with their assistant, re-verifies the pathology report with the picture of the biopsy, and then re-checks the spot on the patient for the fifth time. The whole point here is to ensure the doctor works in the right place, the patient knows what is about to happen, oh, and that you are working in the right place!! "Measure twice, cut once," is an excellent guideline in medicine!

The procedure goes like this:

1)   The medical assistant checks the biopsy against the picture's area, and the pathology report. Then she verifies that the information we have is correct, including the right patient. She also ensures that the patient understands before he signs the procedure consent form.

2)   The provider checks the biopsy picture, area, pathology report, and confirms it is the right patient. The provider asks if the procedure consent form has been understood and signed. Then, the doctor will draw on the area so the patient can confirm the site and understand the extent of the surgery before it begins.

3)   The patient confirms the correct area via sight, a mirror, or a picture if out of direct view. Afterward, the provider asks if the patient understands the reasons for the procedure and if there are any questions.

"Of the people, by the people, for the people" - Abraham Lincoln

4) The assistant then verifies that the site matches the area of the biopsy picture.

5) The provider rechecks biopsy picture, area, and pathology report.

Now, it is still possible to make an incision for the incorrect area, but a lot of errors need to happen along the way! The problem is that about half of patients do not want to do Step 3. They do not want to commit! Patients want their doctors to take *all* the responsibility for their surgery and its outcome. This undeserved faith leads to a complete abdication of responsibility on the part of the patient, which means that this is a very one-sided interaction, and one-sided interactions are not valuable to anyone. A patient-doctor relationship is a relationship, and *no* relationship can be healthy if only one party is responsible and actively engaged in it. Let me say that again: *No relationship* can be healthy unless both parties are equally invested and have similar levels of commitment to shared outcomes.

"Okay, Sam, is the area I drew on the correct location of the biopsy?"

The biopsy was fifteen days prior, smack dab on the tip of his nose, and Sam was in no way, shape or form demented, senile, consuming psychotropic substances, recently kicked in the head by a horse, nor was there any other factor that would make him forget the location of his cancer. Moreover, a scab had formed on his nose. You could see the biopsy site from across the room.

"Hell, I don't know, Doc! That's up to you."

"Well, it is your nose. Does it look like the right spot?"

Now, even if we had a "progressive" Democrat and a "conservative"

"Of the people, by the people, for the people" - Abraham Lincoln

Republican in the room, they would probably have been able to agree it was the right spot, standing twenty feet away. It was obvious. Regardless of how blatant the biopsy was, it's still important to verify the proper location and go through the entire "time out" procedure.

Sam wavered. "We're in trouble if you don't know what you are working on."

Notice how he stops trusting me so quickly? Notice, even more, that he is still unwilling to participate in this encounter or a cooperative patient-doctor relationship? We are about to do surgery on his nose. One would think that he would have a vested interest in finding the correct site so that 1) I could remove cancer from his nose and 2) we would work on the correct area and avoid any needless surgical procedures and 3) we do not sit in the room going back and forth for several hours. To move this in a positive direction, I needed to make a joke out of the situation, allowing him to switch his mindset to something more cooperative, committed, and caring.

"It's not that I don't know what we have planned to do, Sam. We like to get multiple points of confirmation before we get started so we don't work on the wrong kidney today. And you know, if your dermatologist hits a kidney during a procedure, something went wrong," I said with a smile and a mountain of hope that our painful conversation wouldn't drag on.

"If you say that's the spot, Doc."

At this point, it was clear Sam wanted absolutely nothing to do with this procedure. Though we will educate him on expectations throughout the process, along with aftercare and warning signs, he doesn't want to listen. Sam won't read the handout we give to our surgical patients to educate them on post-operative care. He won't watch our free videos on how to care for this incision when he gets home, just like he refused the videos beforehand.

The flip side of the coin is that when complications occur, Sam will not hold himself accountable. He'll never admit that he did not follow instructions. At first, Sam will be adamant that he followed our directions, but when I ask him if he had any questions about the handout, he will claim we never gave him one! That is why he is changing his story about following directions—he didn't have them. We neglected to provide him with a handout! Then, when I ask if he watched the videos, he will say that nobody ever told him about the videos, even though we record all phone conversations with patient consent, and we will listen to the call later to confirm that we did, in fact, tell him about the videos in a documented format.

My point is that at least 50% of the population behaves this way (realistically, it is closer to 85-90%). If you do not, then you might be part of the other 50%, or maybe you did not read the package insert on the new prescription you filled. Maybe, you just scanned the last handout that your doctor gave to you. Maybe, you did not read the consent form; instead, you just signed a piece of paper without knowing what you were getting yourself into because you don't understand the risks, benefits, and options for the procedure.

Physicians are initially psyched to finish training, to get into the real world, and to help people. It only takes about twenty conversations with someone like Sam for a physician to have a real crisis of vocation and wonder how in the world patients can be helped when they don't take responsibility for their health. The disparity is not our fault, and yet, doctors are the only ones held responsible when things go sideways—because the average patient does not have the honesty to admit that he did not care for himself the way he was supposed to, is not actively participating in his care, and is playing Russian roulette with his health. The result is that patients do not get the care they deserve because they are not active participants in their care; they do not get the insurance they should because they do not educate themselves and demand more from the government and the corporations; and the system does not work as it should because it focuses on making money off of disease rather than saving lives through prevention.

Please do not think that our health care system is in crisis solely due to these ubiquitous patient-doctor encounters, yet they are part of the puzzle. Another part is the insanity of insurance companies. The following example took place in an email exchange with one of my billers:

"Dr. Anderson, I finally figured out why we did not get paid for two of patient E.L's visits last year. He was in a skilled nursing facility and did not tell us. Therefore, the approximately $6,000 charge for each of the two visits to you have been denied by insurance."

Let me break this down: about $5,850 of each visit was for a unique type of dressing used to heal chronic wounds. I pay for this dressing and then should get reimbursed for what it cost without making much, if any, profit off it. This is a pass-through transaction, so while I do not lose money, I do not make money on it. Insurance is then supposed to pay $150 to prepare the area, do a minor procedure, and place the dressing on the wound, secure it properly, and then educate the patient. As such, I am out $11,700 from the cost of the dressing alone. I will never get reimbursed. Insurance companies do these types of crooked deals on the new, i.e. expensive, treatments in another effort to deny care and save the insurance company some money. It only takes a few financial hits like this before the average practitioner decides it is unaffordable, and will then stop prescribing the best treatment for the patient in favor of a less efficacious treatment for which the practitioner will get adequate reimbursement.

Tenet 8:
Advancements in health care knowledge and delivery should be encouraged, regardless of profitability.

"He did not tell us that he was in a skilled nursing facility when we asked."

"I know. I told the insurance company that, but they say it is our responsibility to know."

"What if we ask and they deny it?"

"I don't know."

All patients are asked, every single time they make an appointment and when they come into the office, for any changes to their medical history, address, or insurance. Moving into a skilled nursing facility would definitely count as a change. Our questions should have caught the above if the patient was engaged in his care. E.L. was not, and because of his lackadaisical attitude, that's an $11,700 hit, directed at me. It's a bad day, yes, and we have absolutely no recourse. So, instead of making the patient accountable for not letting us know the information and having them pay for just the cost of the material, the doctor must cover it. The result is that patients do not get the best, most up-to-date medical care because physicians simply can't afford to take these hits and still keep the lights on. It is yet another example of the rationing of care that happens behind the scenes in the USA, and it has to stop.

Tenet 9:
Health care needs to be affordable, accessible, and sustainable.

Insurance companies are giants, while doctors and patients are peons. Today, when I prescribed medicine for a patient with Medicaid, the pharmacy would not fill it because it said that we are not an authorized Medicaid provider. This was incorrect, so one of my billing staff members had to spend ninety minutes on the phone with Medicaid, trying to figure out what the glitch was because we have been a Medicaid provider in good standing for years. We are one of the few dermatology clinics in the area to take Medicaid, because it creates these hassles and the pay is atrocious—to the point that most doctors can't afford to treat patients (more discussion on this later).

When Medicaid finally figured out its error, Medicaid was unable to fix it. I had to ask another provider in the practice to send the script from her account because my ability to write a script for Medicaid patients was on hold until Medicaid rectified the situation. The patient finally received the necessary medicine, but all of the extra work for patients with Medicaid is another hit; even *if* Medicaid paid a reasonable rate for services, we would *still* lose money due to the additional time it takes my staff to fix their errors. What's worse—they do not pay enough to cover the overhead. For instance, Medicare will pay $350 for a patient's surgery (note: Medicare rates are a little above the break-even rate for most doctors). And yet, for the same operation, Medicaid will only pay $80—$80! Plus, Medicaid hardly ever pays on time or without hassle, which means it takes extra time for the billing staff to collect, costing even more money. I take Medicaid to help those who need it most, that's the reason why I got into medicine, but we have to limit how many patients we see with Medicaid to balance the costs because, money- and stress-wise, it would make more sense to throw $20 bills out of your car window than to deal with Medicaid. Doctors have hearts. We don't like to see anyone suffering. Insurances, including those like Medicaid, take advantage of this fact. They will deny anything close to breaking even, let alone paying us something for the work. Commercial insurances are just as bad. To afford annual CEO salaries of $17.4 million, insurance companies must play some fascinating games with costs and benefits.[18]

Tenet 10:

Common sense, not overly obtrusive strategy, needs to rule.

Remember the story of the insurance company that would

---

18 "UnitedHealth CEO Makes 298 Times as Much as Its Median Worker." *Bizjournals.Com*, www.bizjournals.com/twincities/news/2018/04/20/unitedhealth-ceo-makes-298-times-as-much-asits.html. Accessed 9 Jan. 2020.

"Of the people, by the people, for the people" - Abraham Lincoln

not spend $4 on medication to keep a fungal infection from eating a patient's scalp? Remember that after we spent an hour on the phone, and the insurance agent hung up on us three times, the patient still had to pay out of pocket for his emergency medication? He was grateful for my efforts, paid for the antifungal treatment, and his scalp improved drastically and quickly. This is not an isolated story. This type of nonsense happens all the time since insurance companies are too big for private doctors or citizens to go after. The government must do more to protect its citizens. This seems to be a common-sense solution: government protecting the citizens instead of protecting the big corporations that pay for whatever legislative bill is passed or trashed.

When you look at the money that was spent in 2018 on lobbyists, it's not hard to see how the law is skewed, how you can buy democracy: Pharmaceuticals/Health Products spent approximately $280 million, Hospitals/Nursing homes spent $100 million, Health Professionals spent $90 million, and Heath Insurance Organizations spent $80 million, which means that these companies spent $460M to make more money from disease![19] No sector of the economy spends more money on lobbying than does the Pharmaceuticals/Health Products section at approximately $4 billion over the last twenty years![20] With all of this money flying around, it's no wonder that, under the Medicare Modernization Act, Congress took away the government's power to negotiate prices for prescription drugs and *Voila!* Americans

---

19 "Health Lobbying Profile." *OpenSecrets*, www.opensecrets.org/federal-lobbying/sectors/summary?cycle=2019&id=H. Accessed 19 Feb. 2019.

20 "Industries." *OpenSecrets*, www.opensecrets.org/federal-lobbying/industries?cycle=a. Accessed 10 Jan. 2020.

"Of the people, by the people, for the people" - Abraham Lincoln

pay more for prescription drugs than any other country—both per capita and in total spending. For the pharmaceutical industry, they got their money's worth with that $4 billion investment in buying laws.

*****

I could go on and on about the daily obstacles doctors face delivering quality medical care, and while a hundred pages of examples from the past year might be a good lesson in realistic expectations in a clinical setting, it would only be mildly entertaining—in a macabre fashion—so we'll return to Sam's story:

With gloves on, needle in hand approaching a very tender nose, I say: "Okay, Sam, I'm going to numb the area now. Please continue to breathe through this and let me know if you need a break. Here we go, ouch ouch." When I inserted the needle into the injection site, he flinched.

"That hurts, Doc."

"Sorry, Sam. Hopefully, that will be the worst part today. Can you tell me if you feel any pain now?" Sam didn't reply. "Sam, can you feel any pain?" Radio silence. Again. "I'm going to start the procedure now. Please, let me know if you feel any pain as we have lots more numbing medicine."

Even when asking for feedback, half of all patients choose not to participate or clue me in if they feel any pain. They won't help me help them.

While I wish this was the exception, these encounters are rampant. Patients do not want responsibility for their health care. It does not matter if we are talking about a surgical site, insurance, prescription medication, diet, or the future of their health. Patients want their doctors to be godlike and powerful while assuming all decision-making power. The problem is magnified when pharmaceutical businesses buy whatever inane law they want—if they throw enough money at it. Insurance companies can do whatever they want because they are too big and powerful to go after; moreover, the system is designed to treat diseases, not prevent them. Doctors have become, through deliberate intention and design over the years, legal drug pushers, not purveyors of some much-needed prevention. Even worse, doctors are the single point of liability in the entire health care equation. When we expect doctors to be and do everything flawlessly, our problems will never be solved; new accountability variables must be introduced to every party involved.

Doctors are not saviors, nor are they omniscient beings who dictate future results. They are resources, but only part of the equation when it comes to your health. It is wrong to assume that individual doctors can do surgery on a system that is fragmented, dismantled, and hemorrhaging on the floor. That is not our purpose. Doctors understand certain avenues to repair the approach to health care in the US, but so do you. You know what it is like to get health insurance, and how difficult it is to navigate these enormous complications. You are part of the answer, and honestly, the most straightforward piece is just trying to take care of yourself so that you do not develop chronic issues. It's paying attention. Still, there is another element that concerns you finding your voice, your power, and tackling these issues on a local and national level. Lobbyists have influenced health care for far too long, and at our expense, because they mostly represent the corporations' interests.

The interests of patients are not ignored. They are entirely forgotten.

Health care is always a major topic of each election cycle, and while politicians spend enormous amounts of time promising the change, they often don't deliver. President Obama came close, but even he, with support in the House and Senate, was not able to pass his preferred bill because the corporations were just too powerful and the citizens of this great country refused to get educated and then get involved. As a result, the passed bill was diluted—a version that could not accomplish everything that he wanted.

Don't get me wrong—I am not saying that either version of the Affordable Care Act would have solved the health care crisis. What I am saying is that even with the bolstering support that was available to President Obama, his bill never passed due to corporate influence. It's highly concerning how much power the top-earning corporations have, and they are dictating our health care policies and daily lives. Their lobbyists make money while the people working within these industries fail to be able to deliver good optimum health care to the constituents.

Nevertheless, these corporations, comprised of people who need health care, should instead invest in sustainable and intelligent health care delivery systems that will help us all live up to our potential. Furthermore, the citizens of our great country need to realize that we have the power to live longer and change laws if we would only care enough to take care of ourselves and hold our government accountable to us, not corporations. If we could do that, we could finally have meaningful conversations about how to achieve it, which would push the needle toward health and away from what we currently have.

CALL TO ACTION

1)   Start doing your job! Read what you are supposed to, seek to understand the procedures, ask questions when you have them, and follow directions for aftercare. Understand your own health insurance and why things are the way they are. Only once you have knowledge will you have the power to stand up for your rights and live a healthy life.

2)   Participate in your health care!

3)   Pay attention to who is trying to buy what in our legislative process and raise your voice.

AFTER ACTION REVIEW

- We have one chapter left, and then you are on your own to research and determine how you will personally get involved. For this chapter, however, you might want to write down what you disagree with and why. Then, please research the issue further to support your opinions.

- Research the pros and cons of lobbyists and write your findings below. Ultimately, it's up to you to decide if our democracy is up for sale and what you want to do about it.

"Of the people, by the people, for the people" - Abraham Lincoln

NOTES:

_____

_____

_____

_____

_____

_____

_____

_____

_____

_____

_____

_____

_____

NOTES:

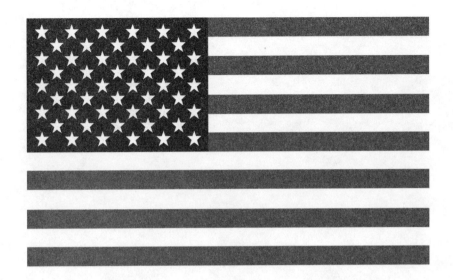

SECTION III

CHAPTER 13

THE PROVIDER WILL NOT SEE YOU NOW

"Let us be the ones who say we do not accept that a child dies every three seconds simply because he does not have the drugs you and I have. Let us be the ones to say we are not satisfied that your place of birth determines your right for life. Let us be outraged, let us be loud, let us be bold."
-Brad Pitt

THROUGHOUT THIS BOOK I have championed the idea of universal health care which, by definition, would be a government-run, or at least a heavily government-influenced, program. For many readers, this might immediately bring to mind the VA health care system ostensibly designed to provide health care for military veterans. That is NOT the model for the universal health care that I would propose. Let me illustrate why, based on my own experience trying to get medical care using the VA system. It will become clear that there are many instructive lessons to be learned from how dysfunctional the VA system is. The VA system needs systemic changes, as does our current health care system in the USA. One is not a valid argument to swing the pendulum all the way to the other side of the equation. There is wisdom in the middle, and if we are honest brokers of personal and public health policy, we can find a solution to a more healthful system. We the people have the power to effect meaningful change if we will just band together and demand—yes, *demand*—better from our elected officials and the bureaucrats who run death care in the USA.

The timing was perfect, I told myself.

Inexperienced, but not naïve, I had preconceived notions about the VA. I read countless articles about how poorly the VA administered health care, and since I had an exercise-induced hernia poking out of my stomach at times throughout the day (that then needed to be pushed back in when it started to ache), I decided to see how the VA system handled something so straightforward. I called to get scheduled. How hard could it be to get an appointment?

It took three months to get a new patient appointment with the VA. My hernia was not that big of a deal—I had already gotten used to pushing it back in multiple times a day—so waiting was uncomfortable, not painful. I wondered what would happen with more severe cases. A month before the appointment, the VA informed me that my assigned provider had decided to take that day off, so we would need to reschedule. Another month passed, but again, it wasn't a stressor. It's not like there was anything really going on.

On the day of my appointment, it was exciting to see the big, beautiful VA building in Colorado Springs. Architecturally stunning, and with a gorgeous view overlooking Pikes Peak, there's nothing else like it in town. There was plenty of parking; the parking lot was never close to full.

"Of the people, by the people, for the people" - Abraham Lincoln

I can't remember the last time I was in a building this nice, I thought, gazing around. It's like something Howard Roark would have been proud of, but if I felt that such beauty foreshadowed a positive, comfortable experience, I was mistaken. Beauty and goodness are not the same.

I found the clinic, ready to check in, but the person behind the desk was busy talking to a colleague. While I did not particularly care about last night's episode of *Real Housewives*, I did not want to be rude or interrupt. After a while, the receptionist looked at me as if I were the one inconveniencing her, then she asked for my name. I told her my last name (it's a HIPAA violation to ask for a patient's full name in an open reception area where others are within earshot).

"Full name?" she blurted out.

I leaned in to tell her my name. Indignantly, she repeated my full name loud enough for everyone to hear, before confirming my date of birth—out loud. While she wasn't shouting, it was high and clear so everyone in the reception area could hear her. HIPAA would have a field day with such sloppy processes.

She gave me some paperwork and asked me to take a seat to complete it. Following a relatively short wait, a medical assistant called me back into the exam area by screaming my full name to the lobby—another HIPAA violation.

Politely, she showed me to a room where I waited twenty minutes for the doctor, but when he entered the room, he headed straight for his computer without shaking my hand. He walked past and took the doctor's chair, not even realizing that I was

"Of the people, by the people, for the people" - Abraham Lincoln

standing. Awkwardly, he realized that he had missed the whole fundamental civility piece. Introducing himself properly, he sat down again and started the long, painful process of fulfilling the same mindless criteria that some bureaucrat in a galaxy far, far away made up.

For forty-five minutes, the doctor hunt-and-pecked the keyboard with three fingers, asking monotonous questions. I reasoned to myself that I could have done all of this while waiting, or the medical assistant could have completed it with me earlier, as her time does not cost as much as the doctor's; that way, the doctor would have been able to avoid most of the tiresome exercise. He didn't pay attention to my answers as he fumbled around dialogue boxes (the same questions kept popping up on his monitor, prompting him to repeat himself over and over again).

Even after I explained that I was a fellow doctor, he forgot that somewhat interesting fact a few minutes later. The entire interrogation was redundant and unnecessary. When the doctor instructed me to hop up on the table, he spent about five minutes examining me and the hernia site, and he sat me down to deliver his plan of care.

He would request blood work, first, and then I would go in for a general surgery consultation.

"Go downstairs. They will do the blood draw." He added that the scheduler would call for the surgical consult within a few days.

"Thank you," I said, and made him shake my hand again, albeit reluctantly, and he walked out of the clinic.

"Of the people, by the people, for the people" - Abraham Lincoln

Tenet 11:

The system cannot tolerate fraud, waste, or the abuse of resources.

The doctor spent about ten minutes doing things that needed his attention, along with another hour performing tasks that a focused individual could have done in fifteen minutes. Being a business owner, I had to wonder how much different my experience would have been if the VA clinic ran like a private practice, rather than a government operation. I looked into it and found that this 76,000-square foot facility that employs over two hundred people saw 25,000 veterans in 2015.[21] Contrast that to my 7,000-square foot facility with less than fifty employees and over 25,000 patient visits in 2015 (many of whom were surgical)! What a difference you can make when you are forced to account for the bills!

I walked downstairs to the lab area and asked the person behind the desk what he thought the anticipated wait time would be. He shook his head.

"Understood. You can't give an exact time, but how long of a wait is it usually?"

"I can't tell you. It might be five minutes. Might be an hour."

"All right. How many people are ahead of me then?"

He pointed to the wall with a sign with a patient number posted on it in white lights, saying, "That's what they're on now."

"And how many phlebotomists do you have?"

---

21 Riley, Rachel. At 2 years old, Colorado Springs VA clinic seeing 30 percent growth. The Gazette. September 25, 2016. Accessed September 7, 2019. https://gazette.com/military/at-years-old-colorado-springs-va-clinic-seeing-percent-patient/article_ff1ff805-e670-57af-9297-fb804aced825.html

"Of the people, by the people, for the people" - Abraham Lincoln

"Uh, don't know," the attendant repeated. "And I can't tell you how long the wait will be. Have a seat. They will call you when they are ready."

"I have another meeting in an hour. All I need to know is if I should come back at another time—or do you think there is a realistic chance that I will finish up in half an hour?"

He shrugged.

At this point, I realized that customer service is a foreign language in the lab, so I sat and waited for about ten minutes when my number pulled up on the screen. A pleasant phlebotomist greeted me, and he was everything a good tech should be: professional, approachable, and proficient. I was impressed by the phlebotomist and I left the VA in plenty of time to get to my next meeting.

Within a few days, the VA scheduler did call, and we tried to find a time to have the initial consult with the general surgeon. The only problem being that the surgeon only sees consults at particular times—in the middle of the day.

After a little back and forth with the scheduler, I asked, "Will the surgeon do a consult at the beginning or the end of the day? It would be hard for me to make a midday appointment."

"No."

"Okay, is there a chance that the doctor could make an exception?" I wondered. "I am a doctor, and I know the procedure that will be done, how they do it, and what is involved. The initial consult would be very quick and easy for him as not as many things will need to be explained."

"I'll check and get back to you," she replied.

"Of the people, by the people, for the people" - Abraham Lincoln

Over the next couple of weeks, I called the schedulers multiple times to try to figure out if they had asked the surgeon if he would consider altering the consult time. I left messages with the original scheduler, and twice when she called back, she only left a message on my voicemail that did not address any of the questions I had, either during the initial call or in succeeding voicemails. Finally, I called and spoke to her supervisor a few days before the system would trigger a new referral (my time was almost up). Apparently, in the VA system, a referral to another specialty only lasts for a couple of weeks, and if the patient doesn't book an appointment, then they're in for another hunt-and-peck-a-thon before another referral can be placed.

The supervisor told me she would check on what was happening and get back in touch with me before the referral expired. She did not. Because of this slip, the next call I received was after the referral expired, and they informed me that I would have to make another appointment with my original doctor to determine if I still had a hernia and still needed surgery.

Amazing news!! I had no idea that hernias could spontaneously resolve frequently enough to necessitate such a policy at the VA (please read this sentence in a tone oozing with sarcasm).

The hernia still forced me to push my intestines back into my stomach frequently. The situation was sad. However, the saddest part is that I couldn't get the care I needed at the VA, and I am a competent doctor who understands how the health care system works. I followed up, frequently, urging them to do their job. Though I have my faculties about me, I could not pry the

"Of the people, by the people, for the people" - Abraham Lincoln

care I needed from the system, and that's when I started thinking about somebody else:

How in the world do people navigate this system? What would happen to someone who is not in the medical field, someone with a disability, someone who does not have ready access to a phone, someone who doesn't know any better—do they have any real chance of getting substantive help? How can we fix this for everyone?

After nine months of refusing to call the VA back to make another appointment, I figured that, since it was time to have my yearly exam, I might as well give it another shot. I called to make an appointment, thinking that my status as an established patient would speed things up. Nope! I was back on a three-month waiting list again.

Fortunately, a few weeks prior to my appointment, I received a letter—a reminder. I also received a voicemail to confirm.

Impressive that they mailed a reminder card and gave me a call to remind me of the upcoming visit. Maybe things have changed! Perhaps there really is a new sheriff in town!

When I arrived at the VA early and tried to check in with the automatic kiosk, it said I did not have an appointment. A very friendly customer service representative was attending the help desk, but she looked me up on the computer, and again, I was not on the schedule. I had the letter with me, and she admitted that she did not know what was wrong, then she suggested that I go to the clinic upstairs. My enthusiasm for meeting the new sheriff had waned—I was not surprised. The only relevant question was, "Will I see a doctor today?"

"Of the people, by the people, for the people" - Abraham Lincoln

When I checked in, there was a pleasant surprise: the receptionist was professional and appropriately asked me to identify myself (in a HIPAA compliant manner).

After a long pause, she looked up to say, "You canceled your appointment two days ago. Uh, so you don't have an appointment any longer."

"I did not cancel my appointment."

"Looks like you received a call that asked you to confirm your appointment or to push a button to cancel. You pushed the button that canceled it."

I shook my head. "I *did* get a call that went straight to voicemail. I never called back because it was a reminder call. There was not an option to cancel the appointment, and I didn't answer the phone, so I did not have an opportunity to cancel the appointment. I still have the message if you want to listen—"

"No, thanks."

"Then why was the appointment canceled? Because I did not cancel it!"

"Don't know."

There was a thirty-second silence, and then the receptionist figured out that, since I was not leaving, she should find a better explanation.

"Would you like to see the letter that confirms today's appointment?" I asked. "Or the voicemail that confirms it? I took the afternoon off work. I expect to be seen today." Another long pause took place where we had a staring contest. She blinked.

"Wait here. Let me see what I can do."

The receptionist knew from my questions, tone of voice, and

body language that I was not leaving without making everyone's job very difficult. She only had two choices: either blame me for their error or try to honor their commitment to deliver quality care. At that time, I was the only person in the waiting room. I figured my chances were decent because absolutely no one else in the department was actually working.

I waited for a couple of minutes, and when the receptionist came back, she said they could see me in forty minutes. I agreed and started to imagine what this process would be like, to be a veteran, suffering from severe mental health issues, and no one to turn to but the VA. It saddened me. Over the course of a half-hour, a few patients checked in and waited, but the clinic was miles from busy.

I see more patients in thirty minutes than this clinic sees in an entire day—with twice the staff and ten times the space!

Later, a door opened, and a VA employee stepped out to yell my full name. *How many HIPAA violations are we counting now?* I thought, stood up, and started walking over to her. Then she called out my name again—I guess I did not jump up and run as quickly as she demanded.

Here we go again, I mused but kept it to myself.

The hallway was empty, and every exam room door was wide open. It was mystifying. Here was a beautiful, giant clinic, and in the middle of the day, nothing was happening. The medical assistant escorted me to the exam room, took my vitals, and re-layed that the doctor would be in soon. While the room lacked windows, it was clean. I waited for about fifteen minutes when the door abruptly swung open.

"Of the people, by the people, for the people" - Abraham Lincoln

Someone barked, "Come across the hall!"

It happened so suddenly that I did not have a chance to see who had given the order. It would seem that in a VA clinic, where we would anticipate a good number of patients have PTSD, it would be preferable to knock on the door and open it smoothly, not burst into the room like Kramer in a *Seinfeld* episode, then magically disappear.

After gathering my things, I stepped into the hallway. I had no idea where the voice came from, so I went down the hall, peeking into random, empty exam rooms until I found him. He never looked at me or shook my hand. He only told me to have a seat. And, like the good dog that I am, I waited for the next barked command.

"I need to get on the computer. I need your name and last four digits of your Social," he said.

I told him, then stared at the wall for about five minutes while he was reading information on the computer. He had still not introduced himself, welcomed me, or even looked over in my general direction.

Then, he looked up at me for the first time and realized, "Actually, you are *Dr. Anderson.*" He paused. "You are a dermatologist, correct?" When I confirmed this statement, the mood of the room changed because I was a doctor—not "just another vet"— and as such, a modicum of respect and some acknowledgment was suddenly due.

Sadness pooled between my ribs, aching for those who did not "deserve" this rare bit of decency. The average veteran would have to deal with this type of neglect and disrespect when he or she could least afford it. With clumsy fingers, he typed in the answers to his questions—some of which were even relevant to the exam, and we identified the next step. While the rest of the exam went well, I hated to think how the rest of the appointment would have proceeded if I was somebody else. I did not even try to get to the VA's surgeon for my hernia. It would need to be done with civilian surgeons, as the likelihood of success in the VA system was slim. This should absolutely not be the case.

Tenet 12:

Public health policy should encourage the entire population—blind to social influences while attentive to educational, regional, and cultural nuances.

Americans celebrate their military when it is convenient. Presidents give us attention when it suits their needs. The military grasps that we have been, and always will be, pawns of the powerful and the privileged; politicians manipulate legions in whichever direction the political winds blow because they don't actually have a dog in this fight—but they sure have position, power, and money riding on it.

Inevitable consequences are integrated into the military lifestyle, along with the cost of defending this great nation. We must accept that. What we can't take is the disingenuous incompetence rife within the government and the VA system. The politicians have blank checks, and with the investment of a new building at sky-high prices, we can see how it pays to send us off to die for a cause in which no one believes. Companies profit when the government gives their Marines shitty equipment, aware that they are treating the military like the disenfranchised members of society, not the responsible soldiers trained to protect America and its interests.

Own it. Don't pretend to care. Don't pretend that you offer excellent services when we are broken and need help. Give us the respect of calling a grenade a grenade. Don't lie and call it a trophy. Or a worthy effort. At least we have earned honesty for our sacrifices. As Americans, it should be easy for us to empathize with those who protect our freedom because these people are real—they are in our families. We can see how unsatisfied they are with the medical system because we live with their frustrations, too.

For those who have lived, breathed, and bled for our nation, the act of supporting such a shambling system like the VA is more insulting than encouraging. I would rather fend for myself and make my own choices than beg for scraps of the VA's attention (when it suits their sensibilities to mind us dogs). Why? Because we are devalued. We have become "other" to them.

Unfortunately, the inefficiencies extend to those delivering the care to veterans. The VA is supposed to offer their beneficiaries access to civilian specialists when they live outside of a forty-mile radius, yet I have heard countless horror stories from VA patients who *eventually* made it into my dermatology clinic to receive the care they needed after they were first denied that necessity. Many, for months on end, were told they needed to drive to see a dermatologist in Denver, which is well beyond the distance limit. Many of them were discouraged from seeing a dermatologist for serious issues, like skin cancer, and many received the wrong treatment for the wrong condition (for months on end); after these poor treatments failed, they had to fight to see a dermatologist. By the time the veterans make it to my clinic, they almost always have a ridiculous story of how difficult it was for them to be seen in their city by the right specialist.

Tenet 13:

We should not sacrifice our rights to implement health care policy.

From the perspective of providers, we should not have to fight for every single thing that needs to be done. There were more times than I care to remember when a procedure, such as a simple biopsy, was not authorized until we went through weeks of paperwork to get approval. More often than not, we need to do the procedure knowing payment is out of the question due to time constraints. If there's the potential for a diagnosis or even treatment, then it's in the best interest of the patient to skip the step of getting a prior authorization, because the service needs to be done now, not in three months when the bureaucrats decide to allow proper medical care to be done. My billing staff spends countless hours trying to get approval from the VA, when every other private insurer we deal with does not require prior authorization for basic services that no insurance should ever question!

Sometimes they pay. Sometimes they don't.

At the town hall meetings, where all the leaders of the local VA were present, I explained how poorly things were functioning and how to improve them. The leaders took down our contact information, promising to get in touch, to fix everything,

"Of the people, by the people, for the people" - Abraham Lincoln

but they never called. The town hall was an assignment—a box to cross off. But an effort to enact real change? Hardly.

At another town hall meeting a year later, I repeated my concerns along with the fact that I'd been rebuffed, and I wasn't the only one—the other audience members were familiar to me. The VA leaders promised that, with the new system roll-out, all our concerns would be solved! When asked how it was going to be different, it was a long walk through a series of nonfunctional ideas. There was no tangible plan. The meeting was nonsense, veiled in pretty, empty promises.

One such promise was that they would have a list of approved procedure codes that would not require prior authorization. After weeks of searching for the list, I finally found the person who could send it over electronically, but when I asked them to clarify the document, they could not. Many terms and procedures described on the list were unheard of in medicine, some were obsolete, outside the standard of care, and some were so vague that I had no idea what they were referencing!

They told me to *trust* them, that everything would be taken care of, that there were no issues to warrant this kind of concern. I offered to help rewrite the guidelines, to simplify precisely, to broadcast the codes so there was no confusion over what we could or could not do. They were not interested. Again, I told them that this document was insufficient. It was either written by dilettantes forty years ago, not a dermatologist, or it was written recently by someone who had no idea what the current standard of care is.

That was not their problem.

"Of the people, by the people, for the people" - Abraham Lincoln

Tenet 14:

Health care is not a partisan issue, and as such, partisan power-plays have no role in the discussion.

The VA system is in such disrepair that I am not sure much other than a complete overhaul by compassionate doctors and a roomful of astute and driven businesspeople could save it (with the backing of Congress). The VA is in the abhorrent business of trying to look good on the outside while doing nothing on the inside to ensure that it's capable of carrying out its mission. The VA will likely continue to be the plaything of politicians hoping to get elected, who then forget as soon as they swear their oath of office.

Medicine follows in much the same way. Health care reform is always in the top three priorities for voters, so that'll get a lot of lip service. President Obama tried his best to pass reform, and regrettably, the diluted bill eventually made things worse. I understand that the forces working against him were formidable and politicians live on compromise. Had the special-interest groups stayed out of it, we could have had the meaningful and positive change that would benefit the whole—not just a part. The health care industry, at around 16-17% of GDP, spends billions in special-interest lobbying to alter the way we run health care as a country. External partisan influence, combined with a patient population that lacks the motivation to care for itself, has led to our current system. It should not be shocking to find we are still stuck with a mess, instead of the sleek, tailored experience that we could have—if those in power were brave enough to tackle the issues, irrespective of any political fallout.

"Of the people, by the people, for the people" - *Abraham Lincoln*

Still, I contend that government-run health care could be efficient...if it were set up for success and fully supported by all involved. It does not have to look like the VA. Let's look at France's health care system, purported to be the best in the world.

1)   In the French universal health care, anyone who resides within the country for more than three months qualifies for coverage. The government then pays for approximately 70% of short-term health care costs and 100% of "costly" or long-term care. If you want to buy private insurance to cover more of the short-term costs, then it is available and more affordable than what we have in the US.

2)   France spends much less on health care per capita and France's system is far superior to that of the US; their advantages include better access to care, more hospital beds, more qualified physicians, more physician consultations per capita, better disease results, longer life expectancy, fewer avoidable deaths, more elderly (living longer is expensive), and there is no gatekeeper for specialists.

3)   Preventative medicine is the foundation of the entire system.

4)   When surveyed, France is more satisfied with their health care system, at 55%, than America—just 28%!22

France's health care system is imperfect. Even the recent strikes show that work needs to be done; nevertheless, their policies are more efficient than ours. If we were to compare Ameri-

---

22 Read from https://wagner.nyu.edu/files/faculty/publications/French.health. system.03.2018%20%281%29.pdf accessed September 7, 2019. Harris Interactive. 2008. France 24/International Herald Tribune, June 2. See Harris Interactive News Room – Western European and U.S. Adults Tear Down this Health Care System!

"Of the people, by the people, for the people" - Abraham Lincoln

can health care with that of Germany, the Netherlands, Spain, and the United Kingdom (all of which are versions of universal health care), then the US would rank lowest in almost every measurable outcome.[23] For the wealthiest, most powerful country in the world, shouldn't we be at the top of the list instead of dead last?

Tenet 15:

Health care policy in the US needs to be constitutionally sound and supported by every branch of the government.

Health care is the primary field where the government can improve the everyday lives of Americans. But what about our current system, Medicare? Isn't Medicare horribly ineffective? Indeed, a government-run insurance program would be inferior to the free-market capitalism represented by private health insurance in the US?! Let's take a look at that because those patients with Medicare need and use, almost by definition, more resources than the younger populations. The older you are, the more doctor visits spot your social calendar.

So, what is Medicare doing well?

1)   Medicare spends about 2% of its total budget on administration costs, whereas the private insurance carriers (like Cigna, United, and Blue Cross/Blue Shield) spend between 12 and 20%! If we switched from private health insurance to a "Medicare for All" system, we would save at least $378 billion

23 Rodwin, Victor. The French healthcare system. World Hospitals and Health Services – Universal Health Coverage (UHC): Making progress toward the 2030 targets. Vol 54 No 1. Accessed September 7, 2019. https://wagner.nyu.edu/files/faculty/publications/French.health.system.03.2018%20%281%29.pdf

a year in administrative costs alone! Some estimates reach as high as $500 billion per year...just in administrative costs.[24]

2)   According to Gallup polls, those with government-sponsored healthcare—military, veterans (ironically enough), Medicare, and Medicaid—are happier with their insurance than are those with private insurance.[25]

3)   In my experience, patients do not complain about Medicare (apart from their insufficient prescription coverage); regardless, prescription coverage needs a complete reassessment within every system. Medicare offers the fewest headaches and places the least-ridiculous demands on my staff when compared to all other insurances accepted by the clinic.

Tenet 16:

Individuals, businesses, and the government should be able to anticipate their health care expenses year after year.

What about business? Wouldn't universal/single-payer health care kill free enterprise in American medicine? According to Warren Buffet, universal health care would help businesses, as Mr. Buffet said that employer-sponsored health care was a "tapeworm of American economic competitiveness." Instead of resting the bureaucratic nightmare of health care on the shoulders of the government, which has the resources to set national

---

24 Manuela Tobias. Comparing administrative costs for private insurance and Medicare. September 20, 2017. Accessed September 7, 2019. https://www.politifact.com/truth-o-meter/statements/2017/sep/20/bernie-sanders/comparing-administrative-costs-private-insurance-a/

25 Riffkin, Rebecca. Americans with Government Health Plans Most Satisfied. November 6, 2015. Accessed September 7, 2019. https://news.gallup.com/poll/186527/americans-government-health-plans-satisfied.aspx

"Of the people, by the people, for the people" - Abraham Lincoln

policy, this burden has been passed down to individual businesses. Then, those administrators must find a way to reinvent the wheel in order to communicate with insurance companies and receive timely payments. It's a struggle. There is no doubt that this wasted time, money, and effort is to the detriment of commerce. Without power or authority, small businesses are at the mercy of large corporations—they cannot make meaningful, substantive changes that would result in a healthier society. If we were to remove this responsibility from individual, small businesses, then they would have the freedom to concentrate their efforts on being profitable (instead of taking over the role of health care administration). They have neither the power nor the authority to do good, efficient work with public health outcomes in mind.

If we look at the history of the industry, going back to the 1960s, health care expenditures were approximately 5% of GDP. Now, they've climbed to around 17%. This stark increase strangles businesses, while also presenting an unfair advantage to our foreign competitors who do not directly pay for their employees' health care insurance.[26] What's worse, American companies have no idea how to budget for their employees' health insurance year to year, as the prices are not fixed; this insecurity also prevents businesses from developing strategies when the cost to deliver health care more than doubles that of inflation.

---

26 La Roch, Julie. Buffett: Medical costs are the tapeworm of American economic competitiveness. Yahoo Finance. May 6, 2017. Accessed September 7, 2019. https://finance.yahoo.com/news/buffett-medical-costs-tapeworm-american-economic-competitiveness-220647855.html

"Of the people, by the people, for the people" - Abraham Lincoln

This insanity must stop.

We have the means to deliver better medicine with lower costs and more predictable outcomes—if we stopped all the rationing of health care and went to a new, universal health care system, where we focus on people, including prevention, set prices, predictable standards, and access.

In its present form, the VA is a disgrace—a model of what happens when the government tries to handle health care delivery, where there is no incentive for them to deliver high-quality medical care efficiently. *No.* Here, the only motivation is to be as inefficient, obnoxious, and obstructionist as possible since their salaries do not depend on performance. They can do atrocious work, pushing people away, and that means less work to do. The VA is, and has been, broken.

Still, we see how the French system works. If health care providers are not good at their craft, then they will have no patients, which means no salary. If they are trustworthy providers, however, then they will have as many patients as they want (without having to worry about a multitude of insurance carriers with different rules and expectations and modes to delay and deny payment). French providers can focus on the delivery of medicine instead of nonsense, with a structure that is predictable, modifiable, and regulated. These factors are switched in the US, and as such, we have some of the worst health outcomes in the world.

*****

"Of the people, by the people, for the people" - Abraham Lincoln

Yes! WE Can!

We are at the end of this book but the beginning of a revolution—one of personal responsibility and action. Commit to your education, involvement, and purpose to help drive this country toward a better health care system, one that is for, by, and of the people.

Perhaps universal health care is not the answer for America, but I think that if we can complete this transformation of personal responsibility and global accountability, it will be the best option. Perhaps I'm wrong. Perhaps you have the better way, but I am willing to listen, then listen some more, and genuinely engage with your ideas, because my ego is not more important than our health.

Join me; let's take back our democracy from the lobbyists, the media, the industries who have the power they have for one reason—because we are not doing our jobs as citizens of this great country. It is time for us to be heard. Join me.

AFTER ACTION REVIEW

- There is just one assignment for the end of the book: consider the spirit upon which this great country was built and ask if we are measuring up...or if we have been found wanting. Then, talk to someone about it. Listen first, then listen some more, then have a dialogue.
- Write down what you learned from this conversation, not what you agree or disagree with, but what you learned.

"Of the people, by the people, for the people" - *Abraham Lincoln*

NOTES:

NOTES:

A *Solution* *To*

Universal Health Care in the Age of Accountability

- Create a system where the tenets discussed in this book are the focal point. Health care, instead of disease care, needs to become the norm. Only in a world in which we care about health more than we care about making money can we thrive as citizens.

- Have a "Medicare For All Who Want It" option that would allow anyone, of any age, to opt into Medicare insurance. You'd still pay the normal, current Medicare tax rate (based on an income percentage) for your Medicare insurance that would automatically start at 65 years of age. There would be an additional charge if you want Medicare coverage prior to 65 years of age. However, your rates would be predicated upon how healthy you are for conditions within your control, not for those things outside of your reasonable control. While the exact formula would need to be worked out, this is the concept:

    1. A healthy 22-year-old person (an individual of proper weight, who exercises regularly, and is a non-

smoker/non-drug abuser) wants Medicare coverage now. He would pay double his normal Medicare tax and receive Medicare coverage now, and in the future (double is because he is paying for coverage now as well as when he reaches 65 years old). His copay, deductibles, prescription coverage, etc. would be the lowest rate available since he is healthy.

2. A 22-year-old healthy person (proper weight, exercises regularly, non-smoker, non-drug abuser) who does not want Medicare coverage now. He would just pay his normal, current Medicare tax for care when he is over 65 years old.

3. A 22-year-old obese smoker, who wants Medicare coverage now. Since he already has two poor habits that will likely cause preventable disease (overeating and smoking), he would pay six times the normal Medicare tax now to cover his current and future costs. The formula would be a multiple of the preventable disease factors. His copay, deductibles, prescription coverage, etc. would be much higher than if he were healthy.

4. A 22-year-old obese smoker, who does not want Medicare coverage now. Since this individual already has two enormous health risks, he would pay three times the normal Medicare tax now to cover the costs of his poor decisions in the future. The actual formula would factor in the number of preventable disease factors and how much those will likely cost to treat in the future.

"Of the people, by the people, for the people" - Abraham Lincoln

5. A 22-year-old person—who is as healthy as they can be given an accident, genetic defect, cancer or other illness that was not caused by poor health choices—would be given the option for Medicare now. He would pay double the normal Medicare tax rate while also receiving Medicare coverage (it would be double, due to the fact that he is paying for coverage now as well as when he is over 65 years old). His copay and deductibles would be the lowest available rate, since he is as healthy as he can be given circumstances outside of his control. If these conditions prevented him from working, then Medicare now and in the future would be free. If this person were not as healthy as he could be given his condition, then his coverage would cost more as outlined in the third example above.

- The above would mandate yearly screenings to determine citizens' health and how much they should pay. If someone considers this an invasion of privacy, they can opt out of the yearly screenings, but that would entail opting out of Medicare coverage altogether—now AND in the future. This would mean that he would need to cover all medical expenses once he hits 65 years of age on.
- Secondary insurance policies would be available from the government as well as private industry to cover all or a portion of what primary Medicare coverage does not. Of course, if someone opts out of Medicare then they can pay for a private insurance policy from private industry. How-

"Of the people, by the people, for the people" - Abraham Lincoln

ever, if someone chooses to opt out of Medicare and private insurance, there will be no free medical care at the ER (or any other place used as a loophole to get free care) as this would constitute fraud, waste, and abuse.

- Health education would be provided, for free, in culturally appropriate ways, to every citizen in this country. If they complete the courses and adjust their lifestyles in meaningful ways that can be measured, tracked, and encouraged, then they will qualify for discounts on their health coverage. A huge part of this would be to educate and encourage proper healthy eating, physical activity, and mental health practices. Prevention will be the focus of the new health care system from birth to death and everywhere between.

    1. Health education and nutrition would start in elementary schools and go all the way through high school, college, and beyond.

    2. Medical schools would be forced to spend as much time on teaching preventative medicine as they do on pharmaceutical intervention.

    3. If people get thirty minutes of exercise, at least five days per week, then they will get a significant discount on their coverage. It would be very easy for patients to track their activity via free apps and other modern technologies.

    4. Processed/junk food would no longer be subsidized by the government. Rather, those foods would have a new tax on them to help subsidize healthier options, which will be made more available to all communities

in the USA (especially places like inner cities where healthful options are sometimes hard to find).

5. Alcohol and tobacco consumption would be tracked, monitored, and taxed. If you think this is an invasion of privacy, then I would argue that making someone else pay for a person's poor health choices is a form of robbery. Also, if you chose not to be tracked and monitored, then that is your right, you just forfeit the right to have Medicare now and in the future.

- Fraud, waste and abuse would be tackled at every level of government and industry.

  1. Laws to limit the monetary influence of lobbyists across all industry must be introduced. Lobbyists can still be present to represent and educate but their activities will be limited to logical, common-sense education instead of buying elections and votes.

  2. The pharmaceutical industry needs to be held accountable for its prices. Medicare must be allowed to negotiate drug prices, which would also mean that we need to determine what is reasonable profit and what is greed, then hold them accountable.

  3. Patients would be held accountable for their choices. If patients are abusing the emergency room, or their providers, or they are "gaming" the system for access to narcotics, or some other form of secondary gain, then they should lose the Medicare option now and pay more for Medicare when they are eligible again at 65 years of age.

"Of the people, by the people, for the people" - Abraham Lincoln

4. Big organizations that have a monopoly on different parts of the system will be discouraged and investigated to make sure that they are not contributing to fraud, waste and abuse. This includes physician organizations like the AMA, "nonprofit" organizations that pay enormous salaries, as well as government organizations that have oversight—no organization is immune and all need continual, independent, third-party investigations to ensure that we are all appropriately utilizing resources.

- Tort reform needs to be taken seriously and addressed on a national level.
- As discussed throughout this book, every part of the health care system would need to be held accountable and take responsibility for its actions. This means transparency of billing, costs of everything, who is gaining from policies, etc.

Each one of these items could fill an entire book; still, the goal is to encourage accountability and responsibility. Each one of the above needs to be thoughtfully considered, vetted, and scrutinized so that we can create a sustainable system that actually works. We need to shift our health care system from Universal Death Care in the Age of Entitlement to Universal Health Care in the Age of Accountability.

Upon these tenets, we will rebuild the "health care" system into something that is of the people, by the people and for the people! **Tenet 1:** Optimal health frees people to secure, on their own

"Of the people, by the people, for the people" - Abraham Lincoln

terms, life, liberty, and the pursuit of happiness. Without health, our potential—both individually and societally—is blunted.

Tenet 2: Increasing the health of individuals will lead to a healthier, whole society.

Tenet 3: While an individual should not be required to make a specified set of healthful choices, each person should take responsibility for the sum of those choices; at the same time, the group should not be penalized for an individual's decision (such as rationing of care and/or resources).

Tenet 4: We need reasonable legal and administrative protections for our providers. We need to advocate for doctors so that they are supported in practicing essential medicine and not the defensive medicine that is also potentially invasive (and costly).

Tenet 5: Every piece of the health care system must be held to account, not just the provider.

Tenet 6: One should have abundant access to resources that promote wholesome choices.

Tenet 7: Disease prevention is the highest priority.

Tenet 8: Advancements in health care knowledge and delivery should be encouraged, regardless of profitability.

Tenet 9: Health care needs to be affordable, accessible, and sustainable.

Tenet 10: Common sense, not overly obtrusive strategy, needs to rule.

Tenet 11: The system cannot tolerate fraud, waste, or the abuse of resources.

Tenet 12: Public health policy should encourage the entire population—blind to social influences while attentive to educational, regional, and cultural nuances.

"Of the people, by the people, for the people" - Abraham Lincoln

Tenet 13: We should not sacrifice our rights to implement health care policy.

Tenet 14: Health care is not a partisan issue, and as such, partisan power-plays have no role in the discussion.

Tenet 15: Health care policy in the US needs to be constitutionally sound and supported by every branch of the government.

Tenet 16: Individuals, businesses, and the government should be able to anticipate their health care expenses year after year.

Together we can!

Together we must!

Together we will!

Semper Fidelis

"Of the people, by the people, for the people" - Abraham Lincoln

ACKNOWLEDGMENTS

Angela, your heart makes me realize how good the world can be.

To my family, thank you for sticking with me through thick and thin.

I want to thank my friends, especially Deven and Steve, who have been so loyal and thoughtful during all my ups and downs.

To my editors Carrie Nyman, Mark, Colin and the Graham Publishing Group, Jeff, Connie, Derrick, and Steve thank you so much for helping me with this book. Your tireless efforts helped bring a voice to experiences and ideas worthy of attention.

To my patients, thank you so much, all of you, for giving me the privilege of trying to help you through whatever ails you. Please know, I am deeply humbled to have been given this honor. This book is one of many steps to provide you with a voice, get you better health care, strengthen our great country, and further honor how amazing you are.

Tony Robbins, you are a beautiful soul who has helped me tremendously. If you have not listened to Tony, do yourself a favor—listen. He will give you the tools so that, if you care enough, you can change your entire world and start living life on your terms and with passion!

And God, even when I turned my back, You had my six. You are loved, and I so appreciate Your love for us all.

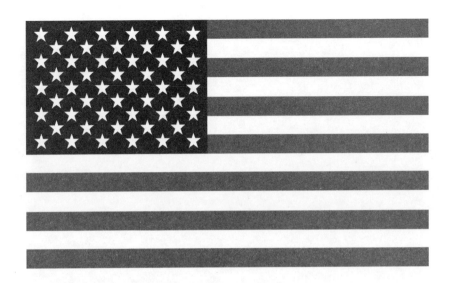

SEMPER FIDELIS